American Disgust

# American Disgust
## RACISM, MICROBIAL MEDICINE, AND THE COLONY WITHIN

*Matthew J. Wolf-Meyer*

 University of Minnesota Press
Minneapolis
London

The University of Minnesota Press gratefully acknowledges the financial assistance provided for the publication of this book by Tampere University's Institute for Advanced Study.

Portions of chapter 5 are adapted from "Normal, Regular, and Standard: Scaling the Body through Fecal Microbial Transplants," *Medical Anthropology Quarterly* 31, no. 3 (2017): 297–314, https://doi.org/10.1111/maq.12328. Portions of chapter 5 are adapted from "Policing Shit; or, Whatever Happened to the Medical Police?" in *The Anthropology of Police,* ed. Kevin Karpiak and William Campbell Garriott (New York: Routledge, 2018), 54–71; reprinted with permission of The Licensor through PLSclear. Portions of chapter 6 are adapted from "Recomposing Kinship," *Feminist Anthropology* 1, no. 2 (2020): 231–47, https://doi.org/10.1002/fea2.12018.

Published by the University of Minnesota Press
111 Third Avenue South, Suite 290
Minneapolis, MN 55401–2520
http://www.upress.umn.edu

ISBN 978-1-5179-1623-7 (hc)
ISBN 978-1-5179-1624-4 (pb)

A Cataloging-in-Publication record for this book is available from the Library of Congress.

Printed on acid-free paper

The University of Minnesota is an equal-opportunity educator and employer.

*For Felix and Ignatius,*
*world-breakers and world-builders in equal measure*

# Contents

# Preface
## THE COLONIAL MULTITUDE

IT WAS WITH SOME PIQUE that I read the recurrent use of the term "colony" in scientific, medical, and popular literature about gastrointestinal disorders and their treatment through the use of fecal microbial transplantation in the early 2010s.[1] Microbial communities, particularly those within the body, were referred to as "good" and "bad" colonies by scientists, physicians, and donor seekers. Donors were assessed for the qualities of their colonies and how they might affect a recipient. People openly wrote about caring for their colonies and providing them with the right kinds of foodstuff through calculated dieting practices. Colonies were "embattled," "under siege," and "thriving." Despite sharing a language that could apply to the historical understanding of colonial politics, microbial colonies exist without politics.[2]

The microbial is as political as the human. *American Disgust* provides a history of our current microbial moment. Tracing the history of the microbial as a therapeutic, *American Disgust* shows how racism has profoundly shaped American medicine at the microscopic level. This has been well established in relationship to genomics, where recurrent ideas about race are applied to genetic code: scholars have shown that what is perceived to be in the genes is better understood as being in the social worlds that individuals and their families inhabit.[3] Type-2 diabetes, hypertension, asthma, cancer—all have social determinants that are largely ignored in favor of genetic explanations. Doing so puts the onus of disease on individuals rather than the societies they exist within. These microscopic politics of blame also shape the microbial, made apparent in discourses about foodways, disease, and lifestyle, all of which are shaped around ideas about bodies and the material they incorporate into themselves through eating.[4]

Colonial politics have shaped the past several hundred years of human society, but their impact on medicine is often ignored. Outside of very specific contexts like medical experimentation in African postcolonies, the Tuskegee Syphilis Study, and leper colonies in the Pacific, American biomedicine has been very successful in dissociating its practice from its colonial origins.[5] Only when controversies arise is attention focused (usually momentarily) on biomedicine's integral relationship to colonialism. On one level, it might be argued that this is all the slippage of metaphoric language and unfounded associations between the colonial practice of medicine as an imperial tool of bodily domination and the way that people discuss microbial communities. But metaphors are sticky.[6] Whether clinicians are actively conceptualizing what they're doing as a colonial practice when they perform a fecal microbial transplant is ultimately less important than that the metaphor continues to dominate how Americans conceptualize the action of bodies on each other. Colonization is invasive; it makes things alike; it displaces what was there in favor of those more powerful. Fecal microbial transplants might be a good form of colonialism, promoting health and remedying life-threatening disorders, but they are inextricable from the medical logic of changing bodies through displacement of one community and its replacement with another.

I started really considering digestion and human microbial communities in 2010. My partner, who was also an anthropologist but who worked in India, was beset with gastrointestinal problems during a period of fieldwork in Bhubaneswar. After a couple agonizing months where her symptoms failed to resolve, I convinced her to come home. Through experimentation, we came to recognize that, if we cut fat out of her diet, her gastrointestinal issues mostly disappeared. At the same time, we went to visit our general practitioner in Ben Lomond, California, who was entirely stumped and referred us to Stanford University Hospital for a specialist. They too were stumped, even after an endoscopy, which revealed no material obstruction, malformation, or disease. At the same time, we were taking advantage of our proximity to Five Branches, a Traditional Chinese Medicine clinic in Santa Cruz. There, her physician prescribed a series of tinctures that we prepared at home alongside his in-clinic acupuncture treatments. During the same period, we were (maybe foolishly) trying to conceive our first child, and (maybe coincidentally) her symptoms disappeared after getting pregnant. It remains a mystery to this day what was actually interfering with her digestion and what solved the problem. But it was a harrowing period of dietary experimentation, medical consultation, and self-monitoring.

She went back to India three months pregnant, feeling healthy. Memory is vague now, but again she had some digestive complaints, which we chalked up to pregnancy. She gave birth to our first child, Felix, a few months later, about six weeks ahead of his due date. Her water broke about seven weeks before he was due, and she spent a week in the maternity ward, pumped up on drugs to delay delivery. She made it a week, reassured by the staff that every day she was able to delay delivery, the better the possible outcomes. Even so, Felix spent two weeks in the neonatal intensive care unit. No one could explain why she went into labor as early as she did, but one of the theories that people were convinced of was that her microbiome had been disturbed by her time in India and this led to an instability in her body's capacity to carry Felix to term. We'll never know. But both of them are healthy now, so we've accepted that whatever was happening was transitory and likely influenced by the complex interplay of my partner's body, her diet, her microbes, and the environment.

These experiences were laminated onto my already food-conscious everyday life. My partner and I have both been vegetarians for decades, and during graduate school—as I ate steamed broccoli over the sink between reading sessions—I committed myself to really learning how to cook so as to fight off the existential experience of eating merely to eat. I wanted eating to be an aesthetic experience. I spent years learning different cuisines through a collection of cookbooks, and even spent a summer teaching in the humanities curriculum at a culinary school, where I learned knife techniques from my students before my classes. Living in Santa Cruz, we were inundated with delicious and readily available produce year round, and I spent time each week at local farmers markets exploring heritage vegetables and other niche produce offerings. Which is all to say that, when we were thrown the curveball of my partner's digestive problems, I was readied with a set of skills and sensibilities to navigate the challenge.

Similarly, when our second child was born with a motor-control disability that interfered with his ability to eat, we were ready with a bank of possibilities that could be experimented with to ensure that we found something that he was both interested in and could eat safely.

Experimentation is key here. In both cases, with my partner and with my child, there was a sense that we could figure something out. With my partner, we experimented by stripping our diets down to their most basic and allergy-free components. From there, we slowly introduced new elements to determine what reactions my partner had, if any. It was through this elimination and experimentation that we were able to figure out that removing fat from her diet would provide at least some kind of cessation to her symptoms. Quite differently, with our child Ignatius, we needed to experiment with texture and bite size. Nothing softer than well-cooked pasta and nothing harder than a corn chip seems to be his comfortable range. But his sweet spot is something like pressed and fried tofu: crisp on the outside and soft and chewy on the inside. The dietician we consulted about his circumstances was basically unhelpful, too focused on nutritious diets and not focused enough on texture; the internet was useless too, as his eating impairment was too idiosyncratic for generic advice to help with it. Only through experimentation could we really figure out what to do.

Desperation is critical too, and it motivated our experimentation. In both cases, we were concerned with the well-being of the family member in question. Not to belabor a point, but not being able to eat is literally a matter of life and death.[7] As is the case with people I discuss later in chapters 5 and 6, not being able to eat leads to immediate and long-term health consequences. Like those people, we were motivated in our experimentation with eating and kinds of food precisely because the vitality of a family member was at stake. Desperation is motivating and it structures experimentation. Desperation provides a way to overcome already settled experiences of common sense about food, bodies, and eating. Desperation is a way through disgust.

Where laboratory experiments might be motivated by the need to prove something and to secure funding and produce publications, experimentation with food for the sake of a loved one's well-being brings an immediate need to experimental practice. Unlike those of the people I describe in this book, our experiments weren't explicitly microbial, but they were all focused on what gets into the body and how. The desperation that characterizes the people I discuss later in the book drives them to much more extreme forms of experimentation, especially using fecal material as the basis of infusions that aim to change their body's microbial colony. This desperation requires them to overcome their disgust related to human excrement and the process of putting it into their body. Their ability to overcome that disgust is predicated on a shifting understanding that excrement is not just waste, but contains microbial constituents that can be harnessed by human bodies. This requires a change in how the microscopic is conceptualized: how the small can become big, how the microbial can become human.[8] If disgust has long been associated with substances, one way around that is to recast those substances as composed of qualities or capacities that exceed previous understandings of the substance. Shit can become medicine through its microbial ingredients, but this requires unsettling disgust.

The story this book tells is precisely about how the microbial was medicine, then became not-medicine. Over time, the microbial would become medicine again, but even so, its status would be contested. The microbial could become therapeutic in its inclusion in foods like kombucha, pickles, kimchi, and yogurt, but that required the transformation of these foods from ethnic to mainstream, from racialized to white. Over the roughly 150 years this book traces, whiteness will be made and remade and remade again, alongside transformations in medicine, food, and everyday life in the United States. Along the way, bodies will be remade too, from permeable and influenced by their environments and foods to isolated physiological machines, and back to environmentally sensitive again. American biomedicine may be on the cusp of a microbial turn in what medicine is, how it acts, and how it conceptualizes bodies. But, then again, it has been on the cusp of a microbial turn for all of its history, and what *American Disgust* shows is that it has turned away from the microbial again and again, preserving particular ideas about bodies, health and disease, their relationships to environments, and biomedicine and its priorities along the way. These forces of preservation are grounded in the affective experiences of American disgust.

# Introduction
## GETTING UNDER THE SURFACE

FOR LUNCH TODAY, I drank a jar's worth of salty-sour lacto-fermented pickle juice. I followed it with two slices of avocado toast, made from avocados and limes imported from Mexico, on sourdough bread baked by an organic baker in our neighborhood, and dressed with Californian olive oil, Indian pepper, and Himalayan salt. I chased it with a small glass of water and a handful of dietary supplements: Vitamin C with citrus bioflavonoids for my tinnitus, glucosamine chondroitin with turmeric for my aging joints, and Omega-3 fish oil for brain health based on a family history of Alzheimer's. This, more or less, is the New American Diet.

If it is more than the New American Diet, it is likely my jar of lacto-fermented pickle juice that is a point of difference. Although lacto-fermented foodstuff—particularly pickles and sauerkraut—have become increasingly available in the United States, they are still an acquired taste. Most pickles in the Standard American Diet are "quick" pickles made from vinegar, salt, and sugar, with a variety of spices thrown in for flavor. Lacto-fermented foods rely on microbes to ferment the vegetables in question, leading to a piquant, umami flavor unlike quick pickles, which are usually sweet and sour. A quick-pickled cucumber might add a little sweetness to a hamburger; a lacto-fermented pickle would add a lofty flavor that plays off the earthy substance of a veggie or meaty burger and its char. If this brief description is palpable to you, it is because you've already acquired these tastes.

But this description may be alien too. Diets are emergent things and are shaped by eaters' socioeconomic positions in the world. The New American Diet appeals to a particular kind of person for whom eating takes on moral and aesthetic experience, often cast through the idiom of "health." As a diet, it stands in distinction to the Standard American Diet,[1] which is routinely depicted by detractors as full of greasy fast food, too many mass-produced carbohydrates, and too few fruits and vegetables. The Standard American Diet is also assumed by its detractors to be bland in taste and monotonous in texture, the materialization of inoffensiveness, unless one is offended by inoffensiveness. Inasmuch as diets claim to be about health, they are also always about distinction: eating certain kinds of food indexes who one is, the status they hold or seek in society, and how they differ from other people. One axis of distinction is "health," where some eaters take their health seriously, while others are accepted as not doing so. Acquiring a taste for the New American Diet is also acquiring the taste for "healthy" eating, which has involved an intensifying interest in the microbial over the course of the twentieth century.

In many respects, this book is about the acquisition of taste. It is about the changing contours of the American diet and how they reflect ideas about health, the human body, and its relationship to the environment. It concerns changing ideas about medicine and their relationship to ideas about race, racism, and kinship. It is about the long arc of American settler colonialism and its effects on ideas about embodiment, healing, and medicine. And, fundamentally, it is about disgust, its basis in the body, the ways it structures relationships between people and between people and their environments, and its role in ideas about personhood and subjectivity. It is a book about experimentation with the self and its nonhuman constituencies through interactions with medicines, environments, and foods that remake the relations between the body's inside and outside, between self and other.

My intent in drinking a jar's worth of pickle juice was twofold. It was, first and foremost, a bit of a dare to myself. I had been teaching my students about autoethnographic descriptions of physiological processes, encouraging them in the context of the coronavirus pandemic to turn their attention to their daily bodily experiences. In getting them to approach these descriptions, I encouraged them to consider how they could change their daily activities in ways to make the familiar strange. How could they change their eating practices to denaturalize their experience of eating? After fishing the last two pickles out of the jar for my children's lunches, I was left with a jar of only juice; what, I wondered, would it be like to drink a jar of pickle juice? Doing so is something that people recommend in many of the online support groups I frequent, all dedicated to the care of one's internal microbial colony. If there was a momentary resistance to the idea, it disappeared with the first sip. I drank the rest in a few briny gulps, no worse for the experiment.

Drinking the pickle juice was also an attempt, albeit fleeting, to experiment with my internal microbial colony. Across the internet support groups, cookbooks, self-help guides, and medical papers I regularly consume, all focused on gut health of one sort or another, there is an interest in developing a sense of interoception,[2] a sense of what is happening inside the body as it digests something. Individuals experiencing a wide variety of health complaints and neurological disorders, from *Clostridium difficile* infection to autism and depression, have taken to experimenting with their microbial communities in an effort to change their physiological experiences. They change their diets and their rhythms of eating and fasting, and they employ experimental medicines like fecal microbial transplants (FMT). These practices aim to change the makeup of one's internal microbial colony, a metaphor that physicians, scientists, and experimentalists use without irony to describe the millions or billions or trillions of tiny microbes that inhabit human skin and organs. Humans cannot know their microbes in any intersubjective way, but they can come to understand them through their reactions to food and medical treatments. Gassy bloat, a rash, being nauseated—each could be the sign of an upset microbial colony. Could I, in drinking this jar of pickle juice, notice a change in my microbial colony?

## Body of Self and Body of Other

Over the course of the eighteenth and nineteenth centuries, the growing traditions of modern medicine and the life and environmental sciences sought to establish the contours of the human body.[3] Where once American medicine and science imagined the body to be relatively porous and able to be contaminated and made sick through proximity to outside forces, especially miasmas, the skin became a barrier between body and environment.[4] This was central to the growing management of human and animal populations in cities, where industrial opportunities for employment drew people into closer proximity with each other and with urban nonhuman animals. This proximity in urban centers led to waves of epidemic disease and the need to manage populations through housing and nascent attempts at public health.[5] Given the absence of the germ theory of disease, only so much could be done, and interventions often targeted individuals symbolically associated with dirt, particularly the working classes. These public health efforts sought to shape individual behaviors, and by extension families, to produce healthy and responsible citizens.[6] Without the germ theory of disease, the focus on individual behaviors and the cleaning of public and private spaces was all that was possible. The management of urban infrastructures, hospitals, workspaces, and schools that would mitigate viral and bacterial infections could occur only after an understanding of how microbes work and how they are transmitted between persons, and between persons and nonhumans.

The skin also became a critical means to distinguish between kinds of bodies, with race being a primary means of categorization and differentiation.[7] The origins of conceptualizations of race mapped onto ideas of kinds of bodies and the diseases they carried in the eighteenth and nineteenth centuries; in the United States, bodies marked as Black, Asian, Indigenous, and Hispanic (although in much different language) were accepted as potential threats to the health of those around them. This included, in an era before contemporary conceptions of whiteness, people of Jewish, Irish, and Mediterranean descent as well. In crowded urban spaces, commingling bodies were seen as a threat; admitting nonwhite bodies into the country was likewise a threat; and the eradication of Native American groups across the continent was taken as preserving and growing the health of the body politic. Racism developed in time to include forms of disgust that grew out of the contact between bodies, nowhere more apparent than in miscegenation laws that restricted sexual contact between white and nonwhite bodies. That disgust was critical for the articulation of whiteness in the United States.

Whiteness is associated with an avoidance of disgust. This is everywhere, from the curation of particular kinds of diets (e.g., the Standard American Diet with its reliance on sweetness and starchy blandness being key), to the management of living spaces and residential patterns, to the contact between bodies, both direct and indirect. As I discuss in the first two chapters, this whiteness was produced through colonial engagements with nonwhite populations and the development of dietary forms of self-management associated with urban—and increasingly suburban—white populations. The form of disgust that it produced was one that was "cultivated": it had to be produced through specific ways of imagining substances and bodies that cast the acquisition of disgust as the development of "civilized" attitudes about one's body, the bodies of others, and social interactions that brought bodies into contact.

Disgust tends to be conceptualized as something inborn, as something that exists in nature and is expressed through our interactions with other people and substances. But I make a distinction between "unsettled" and "cultivated" disgust. Disgust is a real affective response, an expression of negative desire. But it is not universally the same in its expression or experience, and there are significant ways that contexts reshape disgust reactions. Taking a second bite of a sandwich I've already bitten is a different affective experience from choosing to finish a sandwich my child has half-eaten; and both of these are significantly different from finishing a half-eaten sandwich left by a stranger or recovered from a trash bin, as some freegans choose to do. Considering those choices is always inhabiting a "cultivated" sensibility, which depends on making distinctions between the people and substances that have interacted with that sandwich, with some being more knowable and intimate than others. "Unsettled" disgust is unpredictable. Where cultivated disgust relies on distinctions that categorize kinds of relations (self, child, stranger) and attendant risks, unsettled disgust might be cast as more "prediscursive," less predetermined.[8] Can I tell the difference between a sandwich I have bitten and one that a stranger has; do they taste different? They shouldn't, but that we expect they might indexes how categories shape our affective experiences and how those affects shape interactions with other people and the substances they interact with. A fictional sandwich is a benign example, but when categories of people and their practices are subject to the same processes, the effects can be stultifying and lead into the concretization of dominant forms of disgust. One example of this lies in the rise of biomedicine, which developed out of allopathic practices that were cast by their adherents as fundamentally different from homeopathy and other medical traditions that were categorized as too natural and fundamentally uncivilized.

In an era before biomedicine as it is known today, when it was understood as allopathic medicine, the battles for social acceptance and dominance in medicine relied on the distinctions between medical ontologies.[9] Allopathic practice distinguished itself in its earliest iterations by being predicated on the treatment of disease through difference: unlike homeopathy, which treated diseases with medicines accepted as having qualities akin to the diseases they cured, allopathy used medicines that acted through difference. For example, insomnia would be treated by homeopaths with trace amounts of caffeine, where allopathy would treat insomnia with a soporific or sedative. Central to allopathy was the construction of a difference between the natural and the artificial. Disease was "natural," arising either through exposure to natural elements, including bacteria and viruses, and it was meant to be treated by artificially produced chemical agents, elements of a growing pharmaceutical industry.[10] The idea that nature could cure ailments of nature was increasingly associated with nonallopathic medical practices. This was fundamental in changing how practices were incorporated into mainstream medical practice. Proximity to nature meant that a medicine was dangerous, unpredictable, and unruly.[11] Only manufactured medicines and educated physicians could beat out disease through an allopathic materia medica.[12]

One of the results of this professionalization and standardization of American medicine was that medical practices that were associated with particular kinds of racialized individuals and groups were discounted from being medically efficacious. This was critical in delegitimizing both the medicines associated with colonized populations and the healers who employed those medicines.[13] As I discuss in chapter 1, associating the medicines of racialized others with backwardness and bodily risks helped to make stark differences between kinds of people and was fundamental to developing a sense of disgust based upon exposure to the natural. This was critical in developing a sense of whiteness that was predicated on its association with "civilization," cleanliness, and order, obvious both in attempts to "cleanse" the frontier of its Indigenous inhabitants and efforts to clean up urban spaces filled with nonwhite inhabitants.[14] Civilizing through colonization indirectly meant purifying the body of medicines that were based in the natural world, and that may have had microbial elements.

The creation of the modern American body is predicated on the construction of whiteness. Whiteness here is not simply about racial markings, but also about normalcy.[15] In this respect, nonwhite bodies include both those that were explicitly racialized and those that were constructed as being disabled, and in many cases, a set of overlapping assumptions that render racialized bodies into disabled ones. This is most apparent in conceptions of "normal" cognitive functioning that resulted in discourses around nonwhite forms of intelligence that placed nonwhites at lower capacities than white people.[16] But it is also apparent in the medical practices that have developed over the course of the twentieth and early twenty-first centuries that focus on behavioral change. Behaviors that are associated with ethnic or class differences (and this is especially clear in foodways that are associated with type 2 diabetes) are seen by medical professionals as in need of change in order to make healthier patients.[17] This often means counseling patients and their families away from traditional diets and toward ways of eating that approximate aspirational forms of the New American Diet.[18] Similarly, shaping one's sleep to the needs of work and school upholds a form of social normalcy that is associated with whiteness.[19] Being able to work "normal" hours and attend school during the typical school day means being normal and approximating a "respectability" associated with whiteness. In this respect, whiteness is both a state and an aspirational horizon. One can always become whiter.

The converse is also true: one can become less white. This does not occur phenotypically or genetically, although those fears are sometimes expressed, as I discuss in chapter 6. Instead, it occurs at the level of the molecular, in terms of both what constitutes the body and how the body's constitution is expressed through behaviors. In terms of the latter, this is most apparent in the recent use of "noncompliant" to discuss patients and clients and their failures to adopt the behavioral expectations that medical professionals have for them.[20] Not behaving in the ways that are dictated by the institutions that individuals interact with endangers an individual's status in society. This is doubly so for people who are already racialized, disabled, or otherwise discriminated against.

More subtly, there has been a persistent set of discourses in American medicine and foodways that point to the dangers of being associated with particular kinds of medicines and foods: eating the Standard American Diet and using complementary and alternative medicines are all risky. On one level, this is about being compliant with social norms and meeting the standards of everyday behavior that are associated with particular classes of people. On another level, these anxieties reflect the dictum that "you are what you eat." While such a saying is often taken to mean that eating unhealthy foods leads to having an unhealthy body, it always indexes the fear associated with consuming matter that might affect the body in largely imperceptible ways. As I discuss at length in chapter 5, the idea that the body can be fundamentally changed through microbial infusions is a persistent fear, for both medical professionals and individuals experimenting with fecal microbial transplants. Part of that fear is about becoming less white and becoming abnormal.

## Unsettling Disgust

Over the course of the twentieth century, theories of disgust were a recurrent interest of philosophers, psychoanalysts, psychologists, sociologists, and anthropologists.[21] At heart, theorists of disgust exhibited interest in outlining what might be a fundamental aspect of human nature. As a modernist project, the question was whether there was a capacity for disgust that was uniquely human, something that could be said to differentiate humans from nonhumans. As Norbert Elias writes in *The Civilizing Process*,[22] what was considered disgusting changed substantially over time, and a sensitivity to disgust became essential to what was considered civilized. For Elias (and I join him in this), disgust served as a mechanism to separate kinds of people. Although he does not write about the high colonial period of the 1700s and 1800s, it is clear that, throughout this period of intensified colonialism in North America, "natives" are associated with less acute senses of disgust and are relegated to lower civilizational status as a result, as I discuss in chapter 1. This created the foundation for the development of a particular form of American disgust that was based on distancing oneself from "nature" and its disorderly state. Early American disgust depended on associating particular kinds of people with a lack of a capacity for "civilized" disgust, which often entailed a willingness to subject themselves to natural elements that were distasteful if not abjectly disgusting. Nonwhites, which included Black and Indigenous people, as well as ethnic whites, were those associated by early theorists of modern disgust to be willing to expose themselves to nature, if they weren't already living in nature as a sign of their precivilized status. At their worst, early modern theorists of disgust posited that it was precisely because of a racial difference in capacities for disgust that some races were impeded in their ascension to a state of civilization.[23]

Anthropologists, including most importantly Mary Douglas, sought to overturn such an assumption about the linkage between civilization, nature, racial difference, and disgust. For Douglas and those who followed in her wake, disgust was not so much a "natural" function as it was an encultured response to a stimulus that was conditioned by a society's structured sense of order. Societies, Douglas tells us, are highly attuned systems that construct an order, the disorder of which is "dirt." Dirt propels the need of the "positive" act of restoring order through cleaning.[24] These cultural orders are aimed at making the anomalous fit into categories of order and disorder, and at rendering disorder less dangerous through rituals of ablution. Responding to Douglas, William Ian Miller points out that there are certain substances that are naturally repugnant—the sticky, the viscous, the bilious.[25] Such a claim draws from a tradition of thinking about the "abject," those substances that are intimately about the body and its eruptions. For Julia Kristeva, those abject substances were borne primarily from women's bodies, including menstrual blood and vaginal mucus.[26] Such a conception of disgust is based less in an unchanging human nature and more in the construction of kinds of disgust associated with kinds of bodies:[27] particular bodies are subject to forms of discrimination and taboo as an effect of patriarchy, capitalism, white supremacy, and the construction of their bodies and the substances their bodies create as being disgusting.[28] This is evident in the labor history associated with women's bodies on the factory work floor, as well as in the treatment of racialized women's bodies as objects of sexualization and disgust.[29] Disgusting bodies have often compelled Americans in power to contain them.

Rather than accept disgust as unchanging and based in a naturally occurring reaction to particular kinds of stimuli, I argue that disgust serves as a threshold for subjectivity. As a threshold, disgust serves as a mechanism of differentiation. This operates in a set of distinctions between the body and the not-body and runs parallel to conceptions of self and other, the classic distinction that undergirds theories of subjectivity from G. W. F. Hegel through psychoanalysis and poststructural and postcolonial approaches.[30] Across these approaches, captured most clearly in Hegel's parable of the master and slave (despite its ahistorical view of slavery[31]), racism has played a central role in forms of differentiation, described at times as differences between races and at other times as distinctions between ethnicity.[32] These discourses of racist differentiation were often associated with ideas about cleanliness, diseases, and miscegenation and served as ways to police the interactions between bodies, to change bodies to meet social standards of self-presentation, self-restraint, and normal behavior.[33] But if these discourses largely served as mechanisms to keep bodies apart and uphold forms of differentiation that concretized forms of racial superiority, what was less obvious was how substances and their regulations served similar roles.

Blood transfusion and organ transplantation have long been sites of racism and serve as means to demonstrate how disgust adheres in conceptions of bodily substances and parts.[34] Although most American physicians and scientists in the early twentieth century argued for the transferability of blood from one racialized body to another, and likewise the transplantation of an organ from one racialized body to another, the American public was not as convinced. As Susan Lederer discusses, popular representations of organ transplantation traded on racist assumptions about behavior and the ways that a transplanted limb or organ corrupted a previously "decent" white person. Blood, beyond the novel technology of ABO typing that occurred in the early twentieth century, was long accepted as differing between races and ethnicity, with the possibility that a blood transfusion from one kind of person to another might lead to changes in the recipient. Physicians and experimentalists traded on racist stereotypes in their development of novel treatments, including everything from heart to testicle transplants. Yet, if race provided a means of differentiating kinds of bodies through the substances and organs they were composed of, racism also provided the context in which certain bodies could be harvested for white patients, particularly Black and Latino bodies, which served as resources to be harvested with little concern for the personhood of the individual donating an organ.[35] In time, blood and organs became largely exempt from explicit racism, yet the kind of racism they elicited in the twentieth century shares qualities with the forms of disgust associated with fecal microbial transplants and uncommon food-stuff. The "contamination" purported as a danger of being in contact with foreign substances reflects a form of sympathetic magic.

Like homeopathic medicine, sympathetic magic produces similarity in what it acts on.[36] By its very nature, sympathetic magic is "dirty" in this respect because it makes its object like the substance acting on it. In the context of racist associations between kinds of behaviors and kinds of bodies, the possibility that substances carry qualities from one body to another threatens that a person can become less white through the con-sumption of a particular substance, or conversely that others can become more white. At this level of abstraction, this may sound fanciful, but con-sider American dietary recommendations: people who are associated with type 2 diabetes susceptibility based upon race and ethnicity are guided in eating in respectable ways that uphold American bodily norms and di-etary practice.[37] On one level, scientific understandings of nutrients and fats support such recommendations, but these recommendations occur in the context of symbolic associations between kinds of people, kinds of diets, and racialized conceptions of disease. Eating more "white" may also always be eating "healthier."[38] Likewise, eating "ethnic" foods endangers an individual in bringing them potentially closer to particular kinds of disease associated with racialized lifestyles, and which are often read in how bodies present themselves, from oily skin to bodily odors associated with particular kinds of foods or spices.[39] This logic of becoming some-thing different is predicated on deep senses of distinction between kinds of people and what their substances carry—both the substances that come from their bodies and the substances that are put into their bodies.

In each of these cases of differentiation and disgust, a structural rela-tion is held to mark inside and outside, self and other, safe and dangerous. In each case, this depends on some conception of the civilized and the not-civilized: from unilineal conceptions of "savages" and "barbarians," which are colonial understandings of racialized differences that rendered some people "backwards" and "uncivilized," to more contemporary and seemingly less racist discourses of "genetic predisposition" and unhealthiness. If civilized disgust depends on racism, here I want to conceptualize "unsettling disgust" as a process and use it to strategically unsettle "civilized" disgust. Following Marilyn Strathern's ethnographic work with Hagen communities in Papua New Guinea, rather than conceptualize disgust as arising through distinctions associated with being civilized, I want to point to the ways that disgust is always an emergent experience, something that is born unsettled and creates surprising moments of subject formation.[40] Like Miller's discussion of the "flux" of disgust, unsettling disgust highlights how, situationally, something can be disgusting in one moment and not in another,[41] but I want to draw special attention to the politicoeconomic experience of desperation in the context of health care in the United States as a mitigating factor that changes the thresholds of disgust that individuals inhabit. If whiteness is about stasis, control, and homogeneity, then unsettled disgust opens up the possibilities of destabilizing ideas about the body, forms of belonging, and the relationship between bodies and the environments they inhabit.

## Subjectivity, Racism, and Medicine

Racial difference is integral to the formation of subjectivity in the context of American society.[42] This has been the case throughout American history, as differences were drawn between settlers and Indigenous communities, between whites and their Black, Indigenous, and ethnic slaves, and between elite whites and Jewish, Irish, and Mediterranean people. This investment in difference shaped U.S. politics and society and the colonization and development of landscapes. It also shaped American medicine in indelible ways, such as racialized approaches to diseases associated with particular groups and the management of individuals and populations through forms of institutionalization. Fundamentally, the racism of American medicine was based in associations between kinds of persons and the kinds of disorders that they were susceptible to, in terms of both somatic illnesses like sickle cell anemia and mental illnesses like schizophrenia. These associations lead to certain individuals being more likely to be diagnosed with particular disorders as an outgrowth of institutionalized forms of racism in medicine; they also lead individuals to identify with particular kinds of disorders, finding in their descriptions and treatments a logic that aligns them with the institutionalized expectations of their behavior. In this way, medicine provides a foundational set of associations among race, experience, and desirable forms of treatment and care.

This medical foundation of subjectivity is obvious in the historical record when it is associated with race, ethnicity, gender, and sexuality, but it is less obvious when it is associated with whiteness. As discussed above, whiteness serves as an unmarked category and the basis of normalcy.[43] Because of its unmarkedness, associations between disease and the category of whiteness are unmarked as well. But whiteness also works as a categorical inversion. If, as Jonathan Metzl writes, schizophrenia was overwhelmingly associated with blackness in the early twentieth century, then the likelihood of a white patient being diagnosed with schizophrenia was lowered.[44] Similarly, as Keith Wailoo writes, racist assumptions make it less likely that a person of Mediterranean descent with a genetic mutation that leads to sickle cell anemia is diagnosed with the disease than that a Black person with the same mutation will be diagnosed with sickle cell anemia.[45] When whiteness is buttressed with markers like sexuality and class, disorders become associated with those markers rather than with whiteness itself. This is the case with HIV/AIDS and type 2 diabetes, respectively, where homosexuality and being lower class associated individuals with diseases that their racial associations would normally distance them from in American medical imaginations.[46] In this way, whiteness is evasive, as other qualities will always bear the burden of explaining why an individual is susceptible to disease.

Whiteness is also aspirational. Normalcy and whiteness are often isomorphic, with all that is not white being judged on the basis of its variation from the norm of whiteness, as is indexed in discussions of "model minorities" (and minorities generally), and so the desire to act and be white also invokes whiteness. As John Hartigan has argued, whiteness is not an intrinsic quality, but an effect of interactions in "racial situations" that compel individuals and communities to adopt racialized roles in relation to other racialized positions.[47] This is not to suggest that there are not counterpublics that rely on norms that are nonwhite, but rather that the structure of American forms of expertise, as enshrined at least in science, medicine, and law, operates through norms predicated on an obligatory whiteness that is upheld, institutionally and interpersonally, through forms of white supremacy that depend on the promulgation of normalcy and whiteness as two sides of the same coin. To enter into the space of whiteness is to inhabit unmarkedness. To become disordered, to be disabled or ill, disturbs that state of white unmarkedness. In this way, disease, disability, and race are always bundled together.

It is in this context that I am especially interested in the possibilities of unsettling disgust. If American disgust is fundamentally associated with kinds of bodies and their forms of being in the world, with their smells, their substances, the interactional potentials, all predicated on ideas about race, disease, and disability, then bringing disgust to the fore as a set of human experiences is an attempt to disrupt whiteness. Unsettling disgust means purposefully producing the circumstances under which disgust emerges for the purpose of its reflexive experience. In the context of American settler colonialism, unsettling disgust is grounded in the awareness that our affective lives are shaped by the long history of colonialism and racism that have engendered forms of disgust about kinds of people, kinds of substances, and kinds of practices that divide us as kinds of people. My drinking a jar of pickle juice is a modest effort in unsettling my disgust, but there are a variety of everyday human experiences of caring for the self and caring for the other that potentially skirt disgust.[48] American consumerism has led to the progressive alienation of individuals from their bodies and the bodies of others, particular in the context of care.[49] This is most obvious in the case of the care for children, the disabled, and the aged. For those who can and choose to, the care of others has become an industry of strangers supporting family members, from daycare for children to residential homes for disabled and aged family members, and this is made possible through technologies, from infant formula to adult diapers, and the cheapness of care labor. The results of this are that individuals are often made distant from the bodies of those they care about through the mediation of individuals who care for family members. In the United States, this distancing is largely made possible through a political economy that relies on people of color to provide care for disabled or aged family members of white, affluent families.[50] Working through care of the self and the care of others is one route to unsettling disgust, as it provides means to reconceptualize the boundaries of our bodies and the threshold experiences we encounter through our interactions with the bodies of others.

Making disgust more unsettled is a challenge. There are modest opportunities in our everyday lives—trying new foods, consuming certain kinds of media—and from these modest exposures, feeling one's way toward more adventurous horizons becomes possible. American culinary practices enable this kind of adventure for those with the willingness and means, as the consumption of new foods (to you) might unsettle experiences of taste.[51] Similarly, there are means to expose oneself to media of more and less experimental tastes, from *Jackass* to David Cronenberg and Matthew Barney films. These might be banal examples, but they serve as gateways to unsettling subjective experiences and lay the groundwork for reconfiguring one's sense of disgust. Where one goes from there is more complex. Care provision often puts bodies into contact in ways that elicit disgust, but the social organization of care provision distributes bodily contact in ways that protect people from these feelings, as do the technologies that people employ. One possibility is to put oneself into situations where the care for others is integral. But because disgust is a subjective experience, how one goes about unsettling experiences is necessarily individual; in chapter 4, I offer "elimination communication" as a modest example of how this work might be done. As a way into working through disgust and its parameters, throughout this book I offer a series of thresholds that are assays into feeling out disgust and its contours, moving from individual bodies to modes of activism and ending with a discussion of global forms of governance, all of which serve to open up what might be considered disgusting and what we do with those affective experiences to reconstitute ourselves as selves. Where disgust tends to be approached as about bodies and substances, these forays attempt to reconfigure what might provoke disgust, and thereby create new opportunities for experimentation.

## Stewardship and Regulation

One of my motivating interests throughout this book, and specifically in the last two chapters, is the intensification of two forms of social relation, stewardship and regulation. Both are characteristic of a postdisciplinary society in the early twenty-first century,[52] and although they might be construed as being simply about humans and human relations, for me they provide a way to conceptualize human relationships with nonhumans, microbial actors, and structures of governance.[53] Both of these social forms have precedence in U.S. history, and over the course of the first chapters in this book, I establish their grounding in American settler colonialism and their particular expressions in relationship to ideas about race and well-being. At its heart, regulation in the United States is about the construction and preservation of whiteness and white supremacy. Generally, discussions of regulation focus on the market and the goods that move through it. But there are bodies on each end of and throughout these movements, and regulation is often about controlling what reaches which bodies, how that interaction occurs, and what the results are. In the first three chapters, I focus my attention on how the regulation of substances and bodies is integrally about the production of an American whiteness that is counterpoised to ideas of Indigeneity and Blackness. In the final chapters, I focus on how stewardship as a relationship between body and environment serves to uphold ideas about isolated individuals disconnected from their microbial ecologies, thwarting widespread turns to microbial medicine. The underside of stewardship is that it has the potential to dismember whiteness: it has buried within it the seeds of a means to reconceptualize what bodies are and what they do, but bodies need to be taken apart and reconstituted to achieve these potentials.

By "dismembering," I am purposefully invoking an anatomical metaphor that seeks to take apart the white body as it has been constructed through science, medicine, and American settler-colonial capitalism over the last two hundred years. In its place, a more ecological conception of the body can be installed, one that is less attached to the phenotypic and hereditary ideas that undergird understandings of race and is instead focused on the complex sociotechnical environment through which specific bodies are constituted and supported.[54] In chapter 7, as a conclusion, I focus on developing the groundwork for a posthuman environmentalism that situates human and environmental health as coeval and dependent on a medical sensibility that moves beyond individual bodies as the loci of disease and localized landscapes as the objects of degradation. Instead, reconfiguring calls for attention to "planetary health"[55] that have largely developed out of a position of postcolonial whiteness, for the North Atlantic to aid and regulate the Global South, I argue for a situated attention to local human–environmental interactions that promote and sustain communities and their futures as a break from a colonial past and its postcolonial overdetermination. In so doing, I argue for conceptualizing the body as a kind of landscape, coterminous with its environment and the technologies that mediate its relationship with other bodies and the world we inhabit. Conceptualizing our bodies as landscapes erodes their boundaries in favor of a materialist conception of the necessary interdependence of bodies and their environments.

In "dismemberment," I am also interested in taking apart the affective components of American bodies, which I describe in chapters 1–4 as based in sympathy, habit, taste, and disgust. Each of these affects works to create the body as an individualized body, rather than conceptualize it as open to the world in porous ways, which attention to the microbial and its flows through our bodies invites us to consider. Sympathy, or really a lack of sympathy, and taste work to create barriers between people and between people and substances, respectively. Habit and disgust work to instill a sense of difference between people and serve as sites of self-cultivation. The American iterations of each of these affects is particular and is situated within a broader social milieu that relies on conceptions of nature to legitimate practices that are arbitrary and often exclusionary. Dismembering these affects through attention to how they developed, and particularly who aided in their development, works to provide an opening for recomposing the body and its affects in ways that respond to the opportunities and challenges of our present moment.

If the modern period (roughly 1840 through the 1960s) is characterized by a dominant conception of normalcy undergirded by a biopolitics of productivity and social reproduction, as Michel Foucault has written,[56] and it was succeeded by what Giles Deleuze refers to as a "control society" interested more in debt and variable norms,[57] we may be at the precipice of a new set of social relations characterized by the Anthropocene and human–human and human–nonhuman relations. "Regulation" brings together the modernist, state-level interest in the body politic—the management of populations and their productivity, captured in Foucault's discussion of biopower—with the need to regulate the self and its porousness.

But it is also the case that regulation brings together the management of environments through the control of toxic substances and efforts at remediation and wilding, and the management of diets, particularly in the control of foodstuff, agricultural practices, and landscapes.[58] Regulation is about the passage of things (food, microbes, toxins, bodies, etc.) and their control in time and space. To make something "regular" is to impose on it a spatiotemporal rhythm that becomes reliable to the extent that individual lives, communities, societies, and states can depend on its predictable ordering. In the discussion that follows, I argue that regularity in this way is central to the construction of whiteness in the United States over the course of the late nineteenth and early twentieth centuries and that it is readily apparent in how medicine and dietary advice target white bodies and discuss the risks associated with substances construed as dirty and disorderly because of their nonwhite origins.

Disorder and dirt stand in opposition to regulation. Regulation is generally understood as a juridical-economic process and has spawned a diverse body in the economics literature focused on the health of economies through importation and exportation, the movement of bodies through immigration, exposure to toxins through environmentally focused laws, and legal restrictions of financial practices.[59] Regulation, as economists have argued, benefits or harms economies through legal measures. Governments can ease or tighten regulations in response to perceived economic benefits or dangers, but where regulation happens is at the level of the state, whether local, regional, or national. These state regulations have downstream effects on individuals and communities, bodies, and environments. These effects can be both positive and negative, as in the case of removing regulations on pollutants that increase corporate capital production while exposing local populations to toxins that have detrimental effects on health.[60] Regulations on the sale of particular kinds of goods, such as tobacco and other licit and illicit substances, can have beneficial health outcomes.[61] But, in each case, what is regulated, how it is regulated, and the perceived benefits for which regulation is done are contingent cultural and historical decisions and factors that reflect dominant ideas about who can be exposed to what and under what conditions those exposures can occur. How whiteness has been constructed and maintained is, in part, due to the ways that white bodies have been protected from specific substances associated with dirt, disorder, and the racial logics that undergird order and disorder in the United States.

With respect to its contingency, regulation is a politicoeconomic process.[62] This is apparent in the ways that capital seeks "fixes" through regulation. David Harvey advances the conception of the "spatial fix" for the insufficiencies of mid-twentieth-century capitalism, with the appropriation of land and resources as property as a means to generate increasing wealth in the decline of manufacturing in the North Atlantic.[63] The notion of a capital "fix" has been explored in other terrains by Ruth Wilson Gilmore and Julie Guthman, who show, respectively, how the prison-industrial complex and individual consumer bodies serve as fixes for the profit shortfalls of capital in the late twentieth and early twenty-first centuries.[64] In the absence of new surplus labor to appropriate, new forms of profit generation are required, in this case through the intensification of the prison-industrial complex and its production of wages for prison workers and profit from the purchase of land and construction of prisons, and in the case of consumption, through the intensification of consumption around kinds of food, exercise equipment, gym memberships, and athletic clothing. New expenses create new opportunities for capital to "fix" its stagnation, but it requires creating the desire in a society for the expansion of capital into these areas of everyday life. In the case of the prison industry in the United States, extant racism aided the criminalization of wide swaths of the public, particularly those already racialized. In the case of diet and health, long-standing ideas about beauty and fitness associated with whiteness created markets for consumption of particular kinds of goods and practices. Regulation also points to the temporal aspect of these fixes, situating them squarely in the contingent terrain of the politicoeconomic and guided by local expectations of normalcy—rooted in ideas about race, disability, and health.

In the context of regulation, cultural expectations bring together investment in global and local flows of capital, consumption as a social practice, and the visceral experience of bodies in their everyday lives, with particular awareness to the body's boundaries and its integrity. This is most apparent in discourses of "self-regulation," which often focus on ideas about exercise, diet, and health-focused practices. What is implied in these forms of regulation are the temporal experiences of regularity, the ways that spatiotemporal rhythms of everyday life are structured through expectations of orderly and anticipated outcomes. These visceral politics of the body serve as a mechanism to mitigate experiences of risk[65] and take as their focus modes of self-discipline that target one's health,[66] generally through recourse to the immune system,[67] as a means to allay potential breaches of bodily boundaries. In this way, regulatory societies are deeply invested in a politics of becoming[68] that situates individual human lives against the threats that are perceived as endangering their experience of regularity. By extension, regulatory societies are committed to capital's investment in regular, orderly, and anticipated forms of profit generation.[69] Regulatory societies blend bodies across scales,[70] often targeting identified kinds of persons and practices as imperiling the body politic and individual bodies and seeking to control those dangerous bodies through forms of spatiotemporal ordering and standardization.

Across my work, I have theorized the "biology of everyday life" as a way to connect embodied experiences, social obligations and institutions, cultural norms, and environmental forces, all of which are mediated by the others in ways that are irreducible to straightforward explanations of causality.[71] Attending to the biology of everyday life also provides a means to conceptualize how scale operates across kinds of bodies. From microbes, to human bodies, to families, communities, nations, and the globe, regulatory practices scale up, situating the care of one's microbial colony as a similar practice to the management of societies through public health. "Biology" serves as the means by which this occurs, providing a shared substance for practices to target, all of which are construed by those in power to exist in nature, and in some tension with the demands of society and cultural expectations. "Biology" is a discursive production, and what counts as biological in one moment, and what its powers are, changes as a result in alterations of science and politics and their interactions.[72] This has been the case with ideas about race, the effects of diet, and numerous other features of human life, all of which serve as sites for compelling "scientific" tales about human nature that are later troubled. In this context, something like the Standard American Diet, which was once regarded as healthy and based on physiological needs and is now accepted as the reason for poor health among many Americans, serves as a keystone in the management of American society and the way that scale operates in relation to biology in an expansive sense. From dietary advice to medical interventions to school lunch programs to government subsidies for farmers, the Standard American Diet provided a biological basis for decision-making. In so doing, it produced the American body as a particular kind of object that can be acted on in specific ways, as through dietary practice and medicine. As I work toward showing throughout this book, there are other ways to conceptualize the body: I offer the body as landscape as a basis for addressing how the body is more porous than American scientific and lay ideologies would tend to allow.

In the context of the body as landscape, stewardship serves as the means to regulate oneself, one's environment, and the interactions between them. The internally focused effort at microbial management that fecal microbial transplants represent is a kind of stewardship, a management of the self through the control of nonhuman others. Stewardship is also readily apparent in the wealth of diets that have developed to treat gastrointestinal disorders, fasting techniques, and consumer trends around organic and ethically produced foods, which I discuss in chapter 6. Stewardship aims to balance human desires with nonhuman needs, often shaping the effects of nonhuman life in ways that provide positive outcomes for humans.[73] And, critically, stewardship works across scales: it is how the management of microbial colonies motivates the control of environments and their resources in the world at large for human well-being, and, potentially, the well-being of the nonhuman and the environment. In unsettling disgust, practices of stewardship also seek to reconfigure the human, making stewardship central to human interactions with self and other, and thereby implicitly making humans the caretakers of their food-providing environments and the colony within.

## Structure of This Book

This is a book that is largely about other books, or more precisely, other mediated forms of communication about the body. My interest in focusing on the media that I do, such as ethnological studies, medical monographs, self-help guides, cookbooks, and internet support groups, is that, much like the early modern etiquette guides on which Elias focused, these texts instruct individuals on forms of self-regulation. For Elias, self-restraint was critical to the origins of emergent social forms over the early modern period; etiquette guides demonstrated to individuals how to shape their behaviors in ways that met social norms. If self-restraint was focused on the individual self and predicated on the idea that behavior arises internally and needs similarly internal forms of control in the form of restraint, self-regulation is outward focused, seeking to control the exposure of the inside of an individual's body to elements that exist outside of it. The texts that I focus on here tell a story of how self-regulation emerged over the course of the twentieth century, specifically focused on the American diet and dietary advice as forms of medicine, and how, at the turn of the twenty-first century, it pivoted to include the microbial. Self-restraint, a largely human-to-human interactional form, has segued into self-regulation, an interaction between human and nonhuman.

In chapter 1, I focus on John Bourke's *The Scatalogical Rites of All Nations*. Bourke served in the U.S. military during westward expansion in the nineteenth century and served as a liaison to Indigenous communities throughout the Southwest. Amid a life spent writing about military campaigns, Bourke also wrote two early ethnological texts, *The Medicine Men of the Apache* (1892) and *Scatalogical Rites of All Nations* (1891). In the latter text, he draws on his observations of Hopi and Zuñi communities and their use of excrement as a medical therapeutic. He compares their use of excrement to other racialized communities, creating a tale about the ascent into civilization on the part of those societies who have enculturated a sense of disgust that disallows the use of the excremental as medicine. Bourke also offers a counterhistory of anthropology, one that focuses not on exoticized racial difference, but on differences of affective experience. It is these twin elements of his work that I draw on to develop disgust as the basis for conceptualizing the origins of the Standard American Diet, allopathy and biomedicine, and regulation as a function of "civilized," white societies.

Chapter 2 turns to the work of John Harvey Kellogg, particularly his writing on the stomach and digestive processes and his figuration of disgust in relation to particular kinds of foods and the regularity of specific bodily processes. There is a significant literature on Kellogg,[74] especially as he inaugurated elements of the American diet that are with us still, including a heavy emphasis on grains, dietary fiber, and cereal. Significantly less attention has been paid to Kellogg's history of eugenicist thinking, and here I put his discussions of race, diet, and microbial actors into dialogue to show how his conception of disgust is rooted in his understandings of race. I argue that Kellogg's eugenicist thinking and development of disgust is an inflection point in U.S. medicine and dietary practices, and serves as an unmarked influence on how the Standard American Diet and its relationship to race has developed over the twentieth century through biomedicine.

In chapter 3, I turn to the work of nutritionist Adelle Davis, who, over forty years and several books, defined healthy eating in the United States in the early to mid-twentieth century. Working in the shadow of Kellogg, Davis sought to integrate ethnic foodways into the Standard American Diet. Like David Roediger's account of the shifting category of whiteness and its relationship to labor in the United States,[75] Davis is useful to show how foods that were once ethnic—in this case fermented foods like yogurt and kefir—become part of the Standard American Diet; they move from nonwhite foods to white foods. As a case study, I focus on Colombo Yogurt, run by a Boston-local, Armenian, entrepreneurial family in the early twentieth century. Colombo's story and how it is told by the Colombos and the corporations who acquire the company reflect changing ideas about "ethnic" whites in the twentieth century and how their foodstuffs became mainstream, particularly in relationship to discourses about organic, natural, and healthy foods and the cultivation of taste.

Chapter 4 changes directions slightly to focus on children's health, and specifically the use of appetite and bowel movements as a diagnostic tool to know what is occurring inside the body. The chapter draws on parenting guides throughout the twentieth and early twenty-first centuries and finds its foundations in an engagement with Benjamin Spock's "common sense" approach to American parenting. These parenting guides echo, in quite different ways, Kellogg's use of diagnostics to understand what is occurring inside the body and Bourke's discussion of excrement as a kind of augur for premodern societies. Here I am interested in how what goes into a body, what comes out of the body, and when it comes out serve as indexes of what is occurring within the body and serves as a mechanism of diagnosis. These forms of diagnosis move expertise about bodies outside of clinics and into the realm of patients and their families. This movement away from medical expertise and toward self-diagnosis and family diagnosis follows what the internet has provided people: community-based means to ascertain disease and peer-to-peer support for treatment and experimentation.[76] Focusing on diagnosis also provides a way into conceptualizing how risk is known, empirically; the multisensory forms of augury that caregivers bring to the lay diagnosis of illness challenges the reliance on vision as a diagnostic tool in medicine and environmental management. To get to this, I focus on feeding and toileting practices in American parenting guides and argue that nature-based assumptions about children's bodies cast them as transparent containers that can evidence their disorders through derangements in appetite and bowel movements. But to support this, caregivers must develop a form of intimacy that unsettles typical forms of disgust.

Chapter 5 focuses on the exercise of state power on the use of fecal microbial transplants (FMT) through attention to a series of public hearings by the Food and Drug Administration about the anticipated dangers associated with the transplantation of excrement from one body into another. The meetings bring together scientists, entrepreneurs, clinicians, bureaucrats, and one lone patient who advocates for the low-risk, high-reward use of fecal microbial transplants. The challenge, as I discuss, is that, as a medical technology, FMT does more than act on an individual body: it scales from microbial and molecular levels to whole, bounded bodies, to societies, to ecosystems, and vice versa. Unlike pharmaceutical treatments, which implicate bodies in industrial supply chains of chemical procurement and production, FMT implicates bodies in the sociotechnical environments made for them by the societies they are a part of and constituted through. This leads me to a short history of the concept of "medical police," an early public health institution that never succeeds in the United States. This failure, much like the FDA's failure in governing FMT, reflects deep anxieties about nature and society and the limits of what can be governed and how.

Chapter 6 turns to the contemporary moment and the use of internet support groups for the diagnosis and treatment of gastrointestinal disorders, particularly through the use of FMT. I focus on how dangers associated with the microbial are discussed by community members. In many respects, their fears are quite different from those of clinicians and scientists, who are primarily concerned with the transmission of disease. Instead, FMT users, especially those who recruit their own donors and self-administer the solution, narrate concerns about kinship and the interactions of unlike bodies. Their concerns about excremental medicine highlight the lingering role that ideas about racialization and bodies continue to have in the United States, and many of their anxieties are racist in their concerns about different kinds of bodies interacting through the medium of FMT. It is not that the explicit content of FMT disturbs whiteness, but rather that its implicit racialized content makes it dirty and dangerous for patients. I then turn to modern dieting cookbooks that are designed to manage microbial colonies and develop my discussion of stewardship and human health. Drawing on cookbooks that aim to change experiences of gastrointestinal disorder and the groundwork laid in the preceding chapters 4–5 on diagnosis and treatment, I explore how stewardship (the management of the outside to affect the inside) provides a framework to conceptualize how attention to the microbial is changing American understandings of bodies and the relationship between environments and human life. In many respects, cookbooks of the sort that I focus on in this chapter build on a recent turn in cookbooks toward "lifestyle" promotion rather than strict recipe provision, and they posit that real health and well-being depends on an ecological conception of individual bodies and their situation in a relationship with nature that moves beyond standard models of consumption, environmentalism, or medical care. Stewardship is not without its faults. In many ways, stewardship builds on a century or more of environmentalism that has roots in racist associations between people—"noble savages"—and landscapes.[77] But stewardship's ecological conception of life, its environments, and the permeability of bodies to be affected by their interactions with their environments provides a framework to overcome the biases built into American neoliberalism and its focus on individual bodies and consumption as the basis of healthiness.[78]

In chapter 7, which serves as the conclusion, I offer a reflection on the recurring emergence of "planetary health" and attempts to create a planetary health diet. I use this as a way to consider how colonialism continues to shape ideas about diet in avoidance of addressing systemic conditions that threaten individual and global well-being. I then focus on the emerging microbial turn in American biomedicine and how, over the course of the twentieth century, this turn has been initiated and backed away from with some regularity. What makes the contemporary attempt at a microbial turn inaugurated by scientists, health care providers, patients and potential patients, nutritionists and cookbook authors, and environmentalists and other activists different is how broad it is and how rooted it is in an ontological shift toward the microbial. This microbial turn, rather than just being about the incorporation of particular food-stuff in a diet, is aimed at recalibrating the relationship between humans and their environment. This latest microbial turn provides the basis for an ethical recomposition of the world,[79] situating what we eat as a prin-ciple mechanism for care of the future, and offers a substantially differ-ent path from "planetary health." This focus on the microbial builds on longstanding environmental approaches to diet, but in the context of the widespread recognition of anthropogenic climate change and attention to the microbial constituency of human life, the scope of action that stew-ardship provides helps to move between the lives of individuals, their en-vironments, and the globe. Where other forms of environmentalism are vague in their connection between individual action and environmental effects, the microbial turn we are living through is scalar, connecting our necessarily interrelated microbes, diets, and bodies and the landscapes they inhabit. This turn too might fail, ultimately, but it is inflected by this moment of Anthropocene thinking and offers a way forward in un-derstanding what is at stake and how it can be managed by humans and through their relationships with nonhuman others. I also return to my pickle-juice experiment.

In between some chapters are short "thresholds," which move from one topic or historical moment to another through an illustrative exam-ple. Each of these thresholds is brief and seeks to consolidate key ideas from the preceding chapters in advance of forging into the next topical terrain. In each case, I take a moment to point to contemporary currents in scholarship that dovetail with the arguments that I am making and help connect the dots between what might otherwise feel like relatively disconnected points in a 150-year history that moves between settler-colonial accounts of Indigenous rituals and contemporary Facebook support groups for people with intractable gastrointestinal disorders. In each case, I focus on an example that helps me articulate what disgust is and what unsettling it entails. These examples include discussions of Alexis St. Martin, a famous historical medical case, the imposition of whiteness on American diets in food deserts, and the use of FMT to treat life threatening illness. Each moves disgust along a scale, from the personal to the interactional to the social. Such distinctions are relatively spurious, because what I am chasing is how the personal, interactional, and social fold into each other, weaving an affective basis for a subjective sense of disgust that is simultaneously the basis for social organization and political movements. These sections are also "thresholds" because they seek to enact a visceral textualism, a form of evocation that might (possibly) unsettle one's disgust.

Methodologically, this book is undisciplined. In part, it draws on historiographic and archival research on nineteenth and twentieth century ethnological monographs, medical tracts, diet and cookbooks, and parenting guides. It also draws on early twenty-first-century analysis of government, scientific, and medical documents, as well as ethnographic work with online support communities. In doing so, it tells a partial history of American medicine, foodways, and the microbial and seeks to balance kinds of evidence so as to portray the complexities and breadth of this history and its impacts in the present. Narratively, chapters 1–3 span from the late nineteenth through the mid-twentieth centuries, telling how the microbial features in a few representative texts about medicine and food, which set the stage for the late twentieth century emergence of FMT. Chapter 4 roughly narrates the same period, but focuses on parenting as reflective of the broader trends that chapters 1–3 historicize. Chapters 5–7 bring this history into the present and focus on the ways that the historical currents that are reflected in Bourke's, Kellogg's, Davis's, and Spock's work inform the ways that the U.S. government and FMT seekers confront the microbial in emergent ways of conceptualizing the body and its potential for being cured through biological material.

To write about American society is always to write about the dominant, the emergent, and the dormant.[80] To suggest that there is a unitary "American culture" structured by the same assumptions is both a failure to acknowledge how "culture" is never an impermeable container that fails to change over time and a failure to recognize how dominant expectations about bodies, behaviors, and institutions exist in tension with dormant and emergent forms and practices.[81] The Standard and New American Diets are examples of these tensions, and neither of them likely describes how the majority of Americans eat on a day-to-day basis. Instead, the New American Diet is an emergent form, something that many Americans know about and that many may participate in, but it also might be hard to meet its parameters in many small and rural contexts and on many budgets. Similarly, the Standard American Diet is a dominant feature in American society that eaters can participate in and have access to in many contexts, but also might not be desirable for most people most of the time. Instead, most Americans likely eat something influenced by family foodways and shaped by individual tastes, which, because of the multicultural elements of American society, means consumption of a variety of once-ethnic foods that have become mainstreamed through their dissemination and acceptance. In that way, the dominant American diet reflects the variety of foodways that are available to eaters and the idiosyncratic desires individuals bring to those foods. Likewise, medicine, parenting, and forms of governance all articulate differently across contexts and reflect the complex histories that individuals and communities bring to them.

I write about myself throughout this book, as many of the texts, experiences, and modes of practice touch on my personal history. As an experiment in reflexivity and positionality, I try to use my experiences and perspectives as ways into what might be otherwise obscure texts. Those experiences have been shaped by being raised in a relatively secure, middle-class, white, American family. While my father was a physician, he was not a particularly wealthy one, being a poor manager of his finances; my mother, meanwhile, worked part-time as a therapist and worked hard to take care of me and my brother. We were comfortable growing up in the deep reaches of Metro Detroit, which was more country than suburb when we were children. I steered my way through state schools and landed a series of tenure-track or tenured jobs, none of which have paid incredibly well, but all of which have provided enough security to be able to spend money on food—which, if you haven't gathered already, is an important feature in my everyday life. This interest in food was inculcated by my mother, who has long adhered to organic and natural foods, and paralleled my interest in my father's work, which has informed my career as an anthropologist of science and medicine.

It may seem strange to bring together excremental medicine as practiced by Indigenous communities in North America, fecal microbial transplants, yogurt, Kellogg's cereal diet, and American fad diets to conceptualize the microbial and its place in biomedicine, but what they appear to lack in similarities at the level of whole bodies, they share microbially. Each of these substances is about putting the microbial into human bodies, either through mouths or anuses; they are also about taking an expansive environment of interactions and compressing them into food or medicine to affect human bodies. As substances, they are all about the body's porousness and susceptibility to change.[82] Putting these substances together under the rubric of excremental medicine is an experiment in unsettling disgust: can conceptualizing fecal microbial colonies alongside one's breakfast yogurt break through our civilized sensibilities and open up our connections to environments in generative ways?

# Part I
## GENEALOGIES OF AMERICAN DISGUST

# 1

# The Excremental
## SYMPATHETIC MAGIC AND THE UNSYMPATHETIC MEDICINE OF SETTLER COLONIALISM

JOHN G. BOURKE was a colonial man of letters. He rode with General George Crook in the Apache campaigns in the Southwest and wrote accounts of Crook's campaigns of settler pacification and genocide.[1] He served as a liaison with the Zuñi and Navajo in the Four Corners region. He published academic articles in leading journals in anthropology. And he completed a "dissertation," *Scatalogic Rites of All Nations* in 1891.[2] Bourke spent considerable amounts of time among a variety of North American Indigenous groups, largely as they settled into the reservations that had been set aside for them—and they were forced onto—throughout the late nineteenth century. This provided him with a set of comparative experiences that primed him to seek answers to the occurrences that struck him as particularly inscrutable. One such case was that of the Zuñi "urine dance," which set him on the path that would result in *Scatalogic Rites*. But before returning to the urine dance, it is worth considering what Bourke's contributions are and why *Scatalogic Rites* is important to the history of medicine and social thought in the United States.

Writing in the 1890s, Bourke might be considered among the very first anthropologists, concerned, like his peers J. T. Frasier, Emile Durkheim, and Edward Tylor, with the advent of "civilization" and what marked the transition between forms of savagery or barbarism and modern, settler-colonial life in the imperial centers and their frontier peripheries. In this way, he was also a contemporary with early theorists of the American frontier, foremost among them Frederick Jackson Turner, and he followed in the wake of popular accounts of western expansion such as James Fenimore Cooper's Leatherstocking novels. But unlike many of his contemporaries, Bourke had no misconceptions about what life on the reservations and frontier was like; it was rough, unfamiliar, and dangerous for settlers, soldiers, and the Indigenous communities they were displacing. Communities that once thrived were pushed to their breaking points, and part of his responsibilities as an officer in the U.S. military was easing, however he could, the transition to life on the reservation for the communities that American settler colonialism displaced.

Bourke has been with me for as long as I've been working on this project. I no longer know how I discovered his work, but *Scatalogic Rites* has been looming over me ever since I bought a reproduced copy of it. I've mentioned him from time to time, generally in informal settings, and anthropologists and historians who work in the American Southwest know him by name, even if most other anthropologists and historians don't; he's a marginal figure in both disciplines, owing to his career outside of the university. Where others of his generation like Franz Boas were able to commit their labor to the training of anthropologists and the founding of departments that would shape the course of anthropology's development over the course of the twentieth century, Bourke moved from one military post to another, largely staying in the American West for most of his career. Because anthropology has been so small a field, with a handful of people having an outsized effect on the discipline's concerns and forms of engagement, I have sometimes wondered what would have happened to anthropology as a field if Bourke had been more central to its development. His crosscultural, ethnological approach was widely accepted in anthropology, but his interests in white ethnics and the history of groups associated with whiteness were indebted to folklore traditions. His interest in crosscultural approaches was matched by his interest in historical change and continuity, a form of anthropological scholarship that, while problematically committed to a sense of progressive development over time, sought to find common elements in human history. That interest in sameness over alterity runs counter to the early anthropological investment in "culture" as an insurmountable difference between people and communities. Instead, an anthropology of human sameness has the germ of antiracism in it, which makes Bourke's slide into racialized thinking troubling for me.

Bourke is a complicated figure. He is a sympathetic writer, and his account of his sentiments toward the people he is helping to subjugate lacks the paternalism of so much nineteenth-century discourse. Instead, he accepts the Zuñi, Apache, and Navajo as sophisticated, contemporary societies, if not entirely "civilized." At the heart of *Scatalogic Rites* is his sincere desire to understand how excrement is used in ceremonial rituals as a curative and how its apparent employment among the Zuñis in the urine dance has precursors among other societies around the world. His scrutiny of other societies and the role of excrement in their ceremonies is not limited to those that might be thought of "savages" in the nineteenth century. In fact, one of the central concerns that motivates Bourke's imagination is the role of the Feast of Fools in Europe, and particularly among "Aryans."

What Bourke seeks to unravel through his ethnological examination of the use of excrement in ritual is the shared basis of excrement in human magic and, over time, medicine. For Bourke, medicine and magic are intertwined in their shared basis in human excrement. Race becomes important for Bourke because it maps onto the civilized repression of the excremental as such and the replacement of shit with symbolic substitutes that do not inspire the same disgust that shit does, with "shit" being excremental substance that is necessarily abject, as opposed to the more benign "feces" or "excrement." Those "races" or societies or cultures that have successfully moved away from the brute material of excrement to some form of substitute are not incidentally white; whiteness is isomorphic with the ability to conceal the use of excrement through "modern" medicine. As he labors through in his data collection and analysis, all societies follow the same trajectory through sympathetic magic toward a more civilized form of medicine. In that transition, the source of medicine's power is obscured through the repressive tendencies of civilization.

Writing during the long transition between allopathy and biomedicine, in which medical treatments moved from the proprietary, often unregulated forms of snake oil and related materia medica to the industrially produced pharmaceuticals that marked the rise and consolidation of allopathy in U.S. medicine, Bourke provides a framework for understanding the movement away from "savage" medicines and toward industrial, corporate medical production.[3] Medicine in the nineteenth century was marked by a diversity of perspectives in the United States, many of them highly idiosyncratic and associated with particular individuals and schools. Homeopathy, osteopathy, chiropractic, and allopathy all vied for patients, each abiding by a distinct ontology of the body and etiology of disease causation.[4] Allopathy's basis as the foundation of biomedicine depended on a philosophical conception of medicine as based in difference: the treatment should be an inversion of the ailment. Bacterial infections require antibacterials. Viruses call for antivirals. Growing cancer cells require stultifying radiation treatments. Diseases are meant to be starved or otherwise set against an oppositional force—in the form of an industrially produced chemical compound—that will destroy it. This conception of medicine differed from the homeopathic premise that illnesses should be treated with their likenesses or with treatments that share a sympathetic quality with the disease. Excrement as medicine was squarely homeopathic; in allopathy, disease was dirt, as was excrement, and treating disease with its likeness was the opposite of what allopathy called for. Excremental medicine was impossible medicine because it chafed against the presumptions of allopathic medicine, which relied on a presumption of unsympathetic relations.

I write about Bourke and his representation of Indigenous rituals with some trepidation. As Audra Simpson and Kim TallBear write, albeit in quite different contexts, the consumption of Native lifeways by white, settler-colonial readers removes the power of representation from Indigenous producers and writers and often traffics in tropes of the exotic and disappearing Native.[5] To that end, I have tried to include as little as possible of Bourke's description of the Zuñi rites he witnesses, focusing as much as possible on how he represents things, especially his experience of it, rather than that which he claims to be representing. My focus here is on Bourke's interpretation and affective response, which is steeped in colonial disgust. That reaction is deeply rooted in his "civilized" whiteness. How he represents what he refers to as the "urine dance" is a performance of whiteness that situates his sensibilities in relation to the practices of the Zuñi. As a performance, the representation he offers his readers is about the racial situation that he finds himself in as an audience member of the ritual. Moreover, the racial situation that he is in as an author of a text that purports to provide ethnologic data of a foundational set of rituals and religious experiences that are apparent in Zuñi ritual and shared across human societies serves as the basis for a performance of whiteness too. As a white writer myself, engaging with Bourke is also a racial situation, and one through which I find myself articulating my critical approach to settler colonial whiteness: in consuming Bourke as a writer and scholar, it is to vital to foreground his racism and traffic in colonial representations so as to expose how he motivated his role as an agent of civilization and whiteness.

As a text, *Scatalogic Rites* is more nineteenth-century than twentieth. Rather than long chapters composed by Bourke alone, many of the chapters comprise correspondence between Bourke and his contemporaries and long excerpts from published books, journal articles, and unpublished manuscripts. In many cases, Bourke seems to have offered his translation of sources. Chapters are often short and focused on a single topic. Largely, the book is not organized in a logical fashion, and the great middle of the text is arranged seemingly at random, in an effort to bring together a broad swath of evidence that Bourke has assembled. Yet he has a clear introduction and conclusion, and the mass of examples that he has collected adds up to a body of evidence that demonstrates how societies shift away from excremental medicine—and that, for many societies, this transition is incomplete. That incompleteness marks them as existing at a not-yet-modern impasse. Unlike many of his contemporaries though, Bourke does not seem particularly interested in breaking people from their traditions; instead, it seems organic that they will transcend their use of excremental medicine, substituting the excremental with something tamed by civilization.

Race is apparent throughout *Scatalogic Rites,* but in many cases, it seems almost arbitrary that a racialized community is associated with excremental medicine. Bourke, like many of his contemporaries, believed in something approaching a unilineal developmental trajectory for societies, wherein "primitive" practices eventually give way, through rational and deliberate, but also unconscious and symbolic action, to more "civilized" and modern practices. For Bourke, this is captured in the transition of superstitious religions into modern medical practice. Both religious ritual and medical treatments are intended to heal individuals, but the primitive understandings of disease causation and disease itself are fundamentally different from what medicine in the nineteenth century would posit. The rational scrutiny captured in the observational mode of the scientific method would eventually demonstrate how communicable disease is based in viruses and bacteria. Until then, Bourke suggests that the cause of disease and its cure were necessarily clouded by superstitious, irrational beliefs that ascribed disease to the working of gods, spirits, and other supernatural forces,[6] and the cures that were available were likewise steeped in tradition and superstition and relied on convention for their acceptance, rather than their efficacy. In the context of an evolutionary model of social development, there was the need to explain how a practice outlived its utility, as demonstrated by the lack of efficacy. For Bourke and other anthropologists of his era, this could be explained through the existence of "survivals," practices that have continued despite their grounding in now-discredited beliefs.[7] At best, these practices could become the basis for idiosyncratic, "cultural" differences that marked one community as different from another; at worst, they could become distractions from actually efficacious practices, alienating a community and compounding its difference from more dominant communities.[8] In the context of settler colonialism, the prevalence of survivals endangered the grafting of Indigenous communities into the white mainstream. Likewise, the continued use of "primitive" practices by ethnic whites and Blacks in American society differentiated them from those who accepted the growing efficacy of allopathic medicine.

For Bourke, the use of excremental medicine followed a straightforward trajectory. It began with the association between particular kinds of deities and the consumption of excrement to curry their favor. This became staged in specific rituals, both major community events and medical practice. Over time, the actual inclusion of excrement in the ritual gives way to its substitution with less disgusting material; this depends on a growing understanding that the excremental is not just symbolically dangerous, but also has the potential to harm human health. Human excrement might initially give way to the inclusion of nonhuman feces, which in turn facilitates the inclusion of foodstuff made from nonhuman animals as a substitute for their shit. In this way, there is an acknowledgment of the difference in the excremental: "feces" as the scientifically universal byproduct of bodies and "shit" as the symbolically dangerous, transgressive, and abject substance bodies emit. In its final phase, the role of the excremental is entirely sublimated, repressed through the movement in cultural practices away from dirt altogether so that what was once human shit, then animal shit, becomes foodstuff made from that animal in a chain of symbolic substitutions. As a means to disbar the excremental from inclusion in cultural practices, disgust operates to also occlude feces as a medicinal substance, tainting feces with the symbolic valences of shit. This is captured in Bourke's avoidance of even the words associated with the excremental in his reporting.

Key to Bourke's analysis is his role as a civilized subject. He stands in for the reader, who presumably experiences the same disgust that Bourke does as they read his ethnological account. To manage this, he relies on rhetorical obfuscation, omitting words that reference excremental material. In this respect, Bourke also stands in for the repressive functions of civilization, censoring the excremental symbolically while he is simultaneously seeking to excavate its presence in human societies across time and space. As a result, the excremental becomes not just an abject substance that threatens to disrupt the body and its boundaries, but an impossible substance that cannot even be named. This impossibility is captured in Bourke's rhetorical use of phrases like "deeds were committed which the pen dared not describe."[9] Elsewhere he writes, borrowing from colonial tropes of exoticism and racism: "For reasons not ascertained, the use of these revolting medicaments has nearly always been veiled under the language of euphemism. Sheep-dung is rarely called by its own name, but always . . . 'sheep-nanny tea,' etc. In the same manner, the use of human excreta was veiled under the high-sounding designations of 'zibethum,' 'oriental sulphur,' etc."[10] In ascribing the use of "euphemism" to other people, Bourke reproduces the tradition of obscuring the substance he is talking about, simultaneously suggesting that, in the use of euphemism, the people he is borrowing from are civilized too. Again and again, like the people Bourke draws from, he avoids naming what he is describing, affirming that excremental substances are abject in both their substance and their symbolism.

As further example of his squeamishness, consider these excerpts Bourke draws from contemporaneous scholars and correspondence. In each case, the original text omits the term that is being discussed—which might be integral to the analysis—assuming both that a civilized reader can infer what the substance is and that such reader-based inference is

more palatable than providing a clear description. Writing of his correspondence with an interpreter working with a Cheyenne community,
Bourke quotes the interpreter's explanation that, "among the Cheyenne
expressions of contempt is to be found one which recalls the objurgations
of the Bedouins; namely, natsi-viz, or 's—t-mouth.'"[11] That both his cor-
respondent and Bourke feel obligated to render "shit-mouth" in redacted
fashion points to their concern with the sensibilities of their readers and
the abject nature of the word "shit." Similarly, in recounting an ethnological account of Aboriginal communities in Victoria, Bourke writes:
"The Australians believed that if a man did not allow the septum of the
nose to be pierced, he would suffer in the next world. 'As soon as ever
the spirit Egowk left the body, it would be required, as a punishment,
to eat Toorta-gwaunang' (filth not proper for translation)."[12] "Filth not
proper for translation" captures his inability to name the substance being
discussed and the abject nature of the substance in question, unable to become something other than what it is. Finally, writing about Inuit burial
rites, Bourke directly invokes politeness in his quotation of another researcher's account, with politeness echoing the needs of civilized society:

> In describing the funerals of the Eskimo, Gilder says: "The closing
> ceremony was a most touching one. After 'Papa' had returned from
> the grave, Armow went out of doors and brought in a piece of frozen
> something that it is not polite to specify, further than that the dogs
> had entirely done with it, and with it he touched every block of snow
> on a level with the beds of the igloo."[13]

That there is an indeterminacy in what Bourke and the authors he quotes
are actually discussing in each of these passages is a function of both his
civilized rhetoric and the nature of the substances being discussed: their
abject status makes them intrinsically multiple; they could be any number
of substances and contaminate in any number of ways. The paradox of this
elision of the excremental is that Bourke begins the text with an account
of the "urine dance" among the Zuñi that he was stationed with as part of
the American settlement of the Western frontier. In his description of the
event (and its resonances with practices crossculturally), he actively trades
on an expectation that his readers will find the ceremony as disconcerting
as he did.

## The Excremental Ritual and the Religion of Ingestion

This is where it begins for Bourke, his initiation through the "urine dance"; amid a life of experiences among Indigenous communities throughout the shifting terrain of the American West, the urine dance seems to singularly affect him. An element of his disgust is the use of urine in the ceremony, a breach of civilizational standards. But his disgust also seems to be based in dissonance between who he thinks the community around him is and how this particular ceremony disrupts his expectations of the Zuñi as civilized. His writing about Indigenous communities is largely sympathetic, and he treats as peers the Indigenous men he serves with in campaigns against hostile groups in the West. The urine dance punctures his expectations of the Zuñi to the extent that it sets him down the path of ethnological research that *Scatalogic Rites* presents. In the following description of the event, Bourke sets the "clowns" called the Nehue-Cue who participate in the ceremony apart from the rest of the community. He refers to them as "filthy brutes," a rhetorical distancing between himself and the participants, and between the participants from the rest of the community:

> They then squatted upon the ground and consumed with zest large "ollas" full of tea, and dishes of hard tack and sugar. As they were finishing this a squaw entered, carrying an "olla" of urine, of which the filthy brutes drank heartily.
>
> I refused to believe the evidence of my senses, and asked Cushing if that were really human urine. "Why, certainly," replied he, "and here comes more of it." This time it was a large tin pailful, not less than two gallons. I was standing by the squaw as she offered this strange and abominable refreshment. She made a motion with her hand to indicate to me that it was urine, and one of the old men repeated the Spanish word *mear* (to urinate), while my sense of smell demonstrated the trust of their statements.[14]

Beyond "filthy brutes," Bourke's language is freighted with the expectations of civilization: "strange" and "abominable" undergird his inability to "believe the evidence of [his] senses." He literally does not want to believe what he sees, and instead turns to the olfactory as a means to break through his disbelief. Bourke relies on the series of confirmations—the Indigenous woman's gesture, an old man's verbal confirmation, his sense of smell—in order to affirm for the reader that what he sees is what they would see too, and that his sense of disgust is one that they would share, if they inhabited the same civilized affective state.

He goes on, describing the series of events that begin with the drinking of urine and ending with the assurance that, if the events had unfolded elsewhere, the clowns would have eaten human or dog excrement as part of the ceremony:

> The dancers swallowed great draughts, smacked their lips, and, amid the roaring merriment of the spectators, remarked that it was very, very good. The clowns were now upon their mettle, each trying to surpass his neighbors in feats of nastiness. One swallowed a fragment of corn-husk, saying he thought it was very good and better than bread; his vis-à-vis attempted to chew and gulp down a piece of filthy rag. Another expressed regret that the dance had not been held out of doors, in one of the plazas; there they could show what they could do. There they always made it a point of honor to eat the excrement of men and dogs.[15]

Throughout the ceremony, the clowns are experimenting with the gustatory, the olfactory, and the digestive by eating inedible things, and use of the actual material properties of the object (corn husk and rag) and the symbolic qualities of the substances (urine and human and dog shit) to evoke disgust. The clowns describe it as a game of one-upmanship between themselves to demonstrate who can do what, on the edges of human capacity for eating, both in terms of physiological ability and reaction to disgust. The ritual also enacts difference between the clowns and their audience.

Confounded by the ceremony, Bourke seeks answers among the military staff already posted with the Zuñi and the Zuñi themselves. It is explained to him that the ceremony is intended to "inure" the stomachs of community members, presumably preparing them to eat anything they might need to during a period of privation; the ceremony is meant to act medicinally, a prophylaxis against digestive disorder. From there, Bourke comes to understand that the ritual serves as both a religious ceremony and medical practice:

> The *Nehue-Cue* were a Medicine Order, which held these dances from time to time to inure the stomachs of members to any kind of food, no matter how revolting. This statement may seem plausible enough when we understand that religion and medicine, among primitive races, are almost always one and the same thing, or at least so closely intertwined, that it is a matter of difficulty to decide where one begins and the other ends.[16]

This nexus of religion, medicine, disgust, and the excremental becomes the anthropological quandary that grounds his compulsion to understand what he witnessed. The ethnological questions that motivated him were how common the consumption of excrement was among communities around the world and when the exclusion of excrement from these practices occurs, so as to mark a break between primitive and civilized societies.

Confirming that what he witnessed was not a one-time event solely for his benefit, Bourke set about corresponding with his contemporaries. In so doing, he comes to learn that the ritual he was privy to was not singular, either among the Zuñi or crossculturally. Drawing from his correspondence with Daniel W. Lord, who was "investigating the Zuñi," Bourke quotes him as writing:

> One of the Indians brought into the plaza the excrement to be employed, and it was passed from hand to hand and eaten.... They drank urine from a large shallow bowl, and meanwhile kept up a running fire of comments and exclamations among themselves, as if urging one another to drink heartily, which indeed they did.... Some of the sallies of the actors were received with laughter, and others with signs of disgust and repugnance, but not of disapprobation.[17]

As an account, Lord's shares enough with Bourke's to evince a more-than-transitory existence of the ritual, suggesting to Bourke that it had become enough of a tradition that it was at least culturally specific for the Zuñi. Drawing from a letter from Professor Adolph Bandelier, who was working with communities throughout New Mexico, including the Queres, Tehuas, and Tiguas, Bourke quotes that similar ceremonial groups "display a peculiar appetite for what the human body commonly not only rejects, but also ejects. . . . The swallowing of excrements is but a mild performance in comparison to what I have been obliged to see and witness," which included the "sickening obscenity" of watching the consumption of the "fruit in a mother's womb."[18] Taking these accounts as verification that the ritual consumption of excremental material was sufficiently established in the American Southwest, Bourke set about rallying crosscultural evidence of its prevalence and uses. What guides him is the idea that any practice exists along a developmental trajectory and that what he is seeing in communities of the Southwest is a precursor to contemporary forms of medicine, albeit in a more naked and transparent form.

## Sacrifice and the Semiotic Logic of Substitution

Eating shit is symbolically troubling. Setting aside any perceived positive or negative health impacts excrement might have, as a substance, shit is abject. This is because of the ways that shit has been coded as part of the colonial project that Bourke participated in by articulating the excremental as intrinsically related to nature. Bourke's project, implicitly, is to separate the excremental into two substances, feces and shit. The former might have the potential for being something akin to medicine, and Bourke discusses what might be accepted as early conceptions of the microbial and its effects on human health, particularly in relation to foodstuff. But shit is only waste. Both have the potential to evoke disgust, but shit is intrinsically dirty and disordering; it can be employed by clowns for the ritual purposes of unsettling their audience, but ingesting it is not an act of medicine. Coming to understand this, Bourke's construal of the ritual he witnesses is that it is primarily religious in nature. The act of consumption, rather than being for the benefit of the individual (as in the case of medicine), is taken as a benefit to the community, a form of sacrifice of the person in their eating of shit or drinking of urine. He explains this act of sacrifice when he writes that "As a rule, the more painful, costly, unnatural, and disgusting a rite is, the more essentially sacrificial is its character, — for obvious reasons."[19] Understanding this act of consumption as sacrifice leads Bourke to work through the history of sacrifice in religion, focusing on how an act of consumption can bring an individual and community closer to the divine—even when that act is an act of defilement through ingestion of the abject. Fundamentally, Bourke posits that a series of symbolic substitutions takes place to allow for more palatable sacrifices, where one substance is replaced with another that it has a metonymic or mimetic relationship with, "that the part is ever the representative of the whole, and that when the whole cannot be obtained, the part will be equally efficacious."[20] This allows the ritual use of a substance in a limited way that provides the basis for the development of a sympathetic relationship between the divine and its worshippers.

There are, for Bourke, kinds of gods, and those gods demand sacrifices that align with their interests, creating a sympathetic and metonymic relationship between the divine and the substances associated with it. As examples, Bourke writes that "The gods of the Seas had sacrifices of fish; babies were offered to the deities of Childbirth; therefore the gods of the fundament should, naturally, be regaled with excrement and flatulence."[21] Like in homeopathic medicine, there is a sympathetic relationship between a god and its sacrifices: a god is known by its appetites, which reflect its capacities. "Believing, as was believed in their day, that deities ate excrement, why should not they, the representatives of the gods, eat it too? And if a god enter into a man's body to eat excrement, why should not the victim feed him on that which is so acceptable, and by gorging him free himself from pain?"[22] He suggests that humans accepted the ritual consumption of the excremental because of its association with the divine, creating a sympathetic relationship between the eater and the divine origins of the substance.

Godly desire for human sacrifice, in the first instance, is replaced with animal sacrifice, and in turn, whole animals are replaced with their parts, allowing communities to save precious animals while consuming the goods they produce rather than burning them in effigy or letting them rot through symbolic, sympathetic substitution: "As the animal victim became more and more valuable, we have seen that its excreta were offered in its place."[23] As a case in point, Bourke points to India and the consumption of the substances a cow makes in favor of the slaughter of the cow as a form of ritual substitution:

In the early life of the Hindus it is more than likely that the cow or the heifer was slaughtered by the knife or burnt; as population increased in density, domestic cattle became too costly to be offered as a frequent oblation, and on the principle that the part represents the whole, hair, milk, butter, urine, and ordure superseded the slain carcass, while the incinerated excrement was made to do duty as a burnt sacrifice.[24]

That a cow's excrement can be substituted for the cow, itself a substitution for a human, relies on a set of associations that can be transposed from one substance to another. But Bourke is not resolved that each is a substitute for the other, instead understanding in the diversity of sacrifices a set of complementary acts that satiate a variety of demands: "If the cow have displaced a human victim, may it not be within the limits of probability that the ordure and urine of the sacred bovine are substitutes, not only for the complete carcass, but that they symbolize a former use of human excreta?"[25] In this respect, the flesh of the body is of a different symbolic order from the excreta the body produces. In making this split, the effects of consuming flesh can be different from the consumption of the body's products. Building on this assumption, Bourke notes that "the excreta of Christ were believed . . . to have the character of a panacea, as well as generally miraculous properties."[26] In this way, the excremental could be medicinal, but strictly as a religious tool, associating its healing properties not with the substance, but with its origins in the divine.

Of excremental rituals, the ur-ceremony was the Feast of Fools, a holiday that he traces back to the Roman Saturnalia, which resonates with his experience of the urine dance of the Zuñis. Each of these ceremonies, like Carnivale as described by François Rabelais,[27] involved an abeyance of the everyday orderliness of the world where chaos could reign alongside an inversion of normal rules of comportment. In the case of the Feast of Fools, observed throughout Catholic Europe, new clergy were elected to positions where they overrode the standing order of society; the poor were elevated and the wealthy derided.[28] Priests shouted vulgarities, gambled, and ate gluttonously. They dressed as women, danced and sang, and acted like fools. They even, Bourke recounts from a description provided by Rev. Thomas Dudley Fosbroke, "had carts full of ordure which they threw occasionally at the populace."[29] At the end of the festival, social order was restored. Far from being an isolated, idiosyncratic occurrence, Bourke understood the urine dance as providing a glimpse at a long-standing and seemingly universal kind of human ritual in which the disruption of society's order occurs through the deployment of the excremental: "The Feast of Fools would . . . seem to be . . . a reversion to a pre-Christian type of thought dating back to the earliest appearance of the Aryan race in Europe."[30] The existence of the urine dance among the Zuñis was not a sign of backwardness, but rather of a survival that had developed in North America and escaped the repressive forces that led to the disappearance of the Feast of Fools in Europe.

Central to Bourke's conception of change over time are the ways that forces of repression suppress traditional practices that might be locally meaningful. This is especially the case in the context of contact brought about by colonialism and the pressures exerted to control communities and their unsettling activities—which variations on the Feast of Fools might be tokens of because of their shared symbolic bases. On one side, for Bourke, there are the inevitable propensities of human societies that lead them to behave in ways that are nearly universally shared; on the other side are those forces that shape these propensities so as to reduce the risks to society. In the following, assessing the use of substances that induce altered states of consciousness and their role in religious rites, Bourke construes the propensities for a state of disorder as the seat of "primordial religion":

> Two fundamental principles underlie the structure of primordial religion, — Intoxication and Phallism. . . . As human nature feels the necessity of restraint upon the passions as well as a stimulus thereof, it follows that there are to be noted many cases in which a veneration is paid to plants and drugs which have just the opposite effect, — that is to say that where an aphrodisiac is held among the sacred essences or agents its counter or antagonist is held in almost equal esteem.[31]

Bourke understands humans to have certain desires, based in their bodily experiences, and the "restraint" upon these passions serves as the basis for the passions' elevation as religious experience, as well as the substances that affect particular passions. As in his example, an everyday experience such as sexual arousal can become simultaneously desired and repressed. In this way, the underlying function of the Feast of Fools and its variations is to allow desire to be expressed and fulfilled in a contained way that reinforces it. This also allows for the concretization of desire's repression to be made evident and necessary, thereby producing the fundamental structure of repression and the need for self-regulation in "civilized" human societies. He goes on to suggest that:

> This inhibition, under such dire penalties, can have but one meaning. In primitive times the people of India must have been so addicted to the debauchery induced by potions into the composition of which entered poisonous fungi and mistletoe (the mushroom "growing on a tree"), and the effects of such debauchery must have been found so debasing and pernicious, that the priest-rulers were compelled to employ the same maledictions which Moses proved of efficacy in withdrawing the children of Israel from the worship of idols.[32]

Bourke observes the same patterns emerging crossculturally and throughout human history: things that are desired become repressed because, without their "inhibition," they lead to "debauchery" that is "debasing and pernicious"; rulers are compelled, for the sake of their power and the safety of the social order, to restrict access to specific substances and ban the social exhibition of certain practices.

Discussing the Feast of Fools specifically, Bourke writes that a symbolic substitution likely occurred: "In twelve to fifteen hundred years the rite might have been well sublimed from the eating of pure excrement, as among the Zuñis, to the consumption of the *boudin,* the excrement symbol," which Bourke explains in a footnote as also being "very probably a phallic symbol also."[33] The excremental symbol serves both to represent the excremental sacrifice and to index the sexual desire repressed by everyday inhibitions. The boudin, the sausage, makes the divine an everyday experience through its conversion from a piece of shit into an everyday foodstuff. Elsewhere, noting the historical segue of religious into medical practices, Bourke writes:

Father Le Jeune must have been on the track of something corresponding to an ur-orgy among the Hurons when he learned that the
devil imposed upon the sick, in dreams, the duty of wallowing in ordure if they hoped for restoration to health. This penitential wallowing was retained by nations of a high order of advancement, the ordure of primitive times being generally superseded by clay and other
less filthy matter.[34]

Even while a ritual may remain largely intact, changing understandings of
feces and shit drive the substitution of one substance for another, resulting, for many societies, in traditions that seem to bear no resemblance to
the Feast of Fools and its variations, hence how mud and clay can substitute for excrement. Yet, at root, they are the same ceremonial enactment
of defilement and upset social order.

   The question that remains for Bourke is why, despite both a symbolic ban on the consumption of shit and the recognition that feces is
not medicinal, some individuals and communities continue the practice
of its consumption. He accepts that the only likely possibilities for the
continued use of excrement is a function of "perverted cerebration" and
that there is a fundamental connection between altered consciousness
and religion:

   [The] prophet [Ezekiel] unquestionably was influenced and actuated
   by the ideas of his day and generation, which looked upon the humil-
   iations to which he subjected himself as the outward manifestations
   of an inward spirituality.
      Psychologically speaking, there is no great difference between the
   consumption of human excrement and the act of lying on one's side
   for three hundred and ninety days [Ezekiel 4:4–17]; both are indi-
   cations of the same perverted cerebration, mistaken with such frequency for piety and holiness.[35]

Bourke reaches this perspective by working through Ezekiel's trial, in
which he was told to make bread of "wheat and barley, beans and lentils,
millet and spelt" and then bake it over a fire of human dung, and that
the substitution of cow dung is allowed when Ezekiel protests, thereby
evincing his civilized status. Bourke goes on to suggest that, within the

repressive confines of "civilization," the only likely explanations for the consumption of excrement are "mania" and "abnormal appetite," both of which allow for the possibility of excremental rituals, but situate them as pathological and individualized in some way and not part of "civilized" society; they might, however, continue to exist in just the way that the Feast of Fools did—as an inversion of the normal organization of society and its mores.

> So long as the lines of investigation are included within civilized lim-
> its, the instances [of excremental rituals] noticed very properly fall
> under the classification of mania and abnormal appetite; and the lat-
> ter, in turn, may be subdivided into the two classes of the innate and
> the acquired, the second of which has presented a constant decrease
> since the physicians have rejected such disgusting remedial agents
> from the Materia Medica.[36]

The use of "innate and acquired" here indexes how a practice like the ritual use of excrement could continue despite all efforts to discredit or ban its use. As an "acquired" practice, it could become a survival, and one that potentially finds new functions as its use continues into new social contexts. From its initial religious use, the excremental segues into medical practice, its association with curatives intact. To that end, Bourke suggests that "mankind accepts and complies with ritualistic precepts without inquiry, and even with a vague belief that the more archaic a practice may be, the more efficacy it must necessarily have in securing protection and good fortune."[37] Whereas some colonial observers might have construed the continued practice of the urine dance (and other variations of the Feast of Fools) as a function of the backwardness of particular races, Bourke argues that it is merely a function of culture and uninterrogated practices that allows a community to continue to practice a set of otherwise "disgusting" acts and uses of excrement. That a community might continue to hold onto the vestiges of an excremental practice marks their distinction from those civilized communities who have left the excremental behind or converted it into the basis of a symbolic, ritual practice.

The articulation of sympathetic magic against an unsympathetic medicine is critical in the development of American attitudes about medicine and the body. Inasmuch as "sympathy" is an ascribed quality of substances and their actions on human bodies, it also serves as a way to structure how people want to interact with substances. If we imagine that a substance will make us like it or share qualities with it, how we interact with that substance will necessarily change. Developing a sense of disgust as protective and as a form of being unsympathetic supports the articulation of allopathic medicine's distinctiveness from other colonial medical practices; it also constructs allopathy as a particular kind of colonial practice that acts on the body by colonizing it with difference rather than sameness, as homeopathy would. That this development of lack of sympathy is racially coded is not incidental, but serves to position the body of Americans as mediating between medicinal substances and society. In being positioned in this way, the body becomes the site of managing risks, which a sense of unsympathy supports—and which maps onto ideas about racial difference.

## Racial Maps of Disgust

For Bourke, as for many of the people he draws on for his evidence and argumentation, races are distinct physiognomic types associated with specific geographic areas. Among these racial groups, Aryans exist as prototypically white, but also as the basis for groups around the world whose ancestry seems to demonstrate a shared geographical and physiognomic stock through linguistics and migration patterns.[38] For example, Bourke writes:

> Taking into consideration the fact that these people [Buddhist monks in Tibet], although remotely, are related to the Aryan stock, which is the ancestor of English, German, Irish, Latin, and others, from which we spring, the meaning [of *pedung*], as here given, is certainly not without significance. "Dung," in our own tongue, means nothing more or less than remains, reliquiae of a certain kind.[39]

Tibetan monks become associated with Aryans through linguistic forms and ceremonial practices tied together through a shared archaic relation. Whereas "the use of human and animal egestae in religious ceremonial was common all over the world, antedating the Roman Saturnalia, or at least totally unconnected with it,"[40] attention to the specificities of particular communities can reveal linkages to demonstrate how a shared history gives way to a variety of social forms, all of which incline toward a set of civilized practices that, while acting against disgust, are also predicated on it.

If Aryans provide Bourke with a European race that grounds the basis for civilization, they stand in contrast to many of the races associated with colonial spaces, especially Africa and the Pacific. To draw these distinctions, he relies heavily on colonial ethnographic and ethnologic accounts of colonial officers, missionaries, and early anthropologists, many of whom he directly corresponds with. In many cases, the accounts Bourke draws on are explicitly racist, associating communities and their practices with innate and enduring forms of difference that are explained by racialized capacities associated with fundamental natural differences. Writing about the Aboriginal communities of Australia with the troubling phrase "our blacks," John Frazer conveys that the use of excrement in ritual continues despite the forces of British colonialism:

> Various considerations, however, lead me to think it possible that our blacks, in some places at least (for their observances are not everywhere the same), may use ordure and urine in that way, thinking that the evil spirit will be propitiated by their eating in his honor that which he himself delights to eat; just as in Northwestern India a devotee may be seen going about with his body plastered all over with human dung in honor of his god. And our blacks have good reason to try to propitiate this unclean spirit (Gunung-dhukhya) in every possible way, for they believe that he can enter their bodies, and effecting a lodgment in their abdomen, feed there on the foulest of the contents, and thus cause cramps, fits, madness, and other serious disorders.[41]

Frazer, like Bourke, invokes a colonial analogy between one nonwhite community and another, employing such an association to distance the Indigenous communities of Australia and India from their white colonizers.

Surveying ethnologic accounts, Bourke uncovers other occurrences of the continued use of excrement in ritual and daily practice, in each case implicitly relying on the blackness of a community as explanatory of their difference from their white colonizers. Of the Dinka of East Africa, he quotes ethnologist Georg August Schweinfurth: "Every idea and thought of the Dinka is how to acquire and maintain cattle; a certain kind of reverence would seem to be paid them; even their offal is considered of high importance. The dung, which is burnt to ashes for sleeping in and for smearing their persons, and the urine, which is used for washing and as a substitute for salt, are their daily requisites."[42] Similarly, drawing from Verney Lovett Cameron's account of his trip across central Africa, Bourke writes that "Cameron employed a native medicine-man, near Lake Tanganyika, to treat one of his men who had injured his eye. 'His treatment consisted of a plaster of mud and dirt, and his fee was forty strings of beads.'" Bourke writes in a footnote: "The word 'dirt,' as used by Cameron, . . . no doubt means ordure."[43] As an inverted image of Europe, Africa provides Bourke and his contemporaries with a foil to the mores of the civilized, colonial powers. At the edges of Bourke's thought, it becomes apparent how these views of Black communities informed his contextualization of his experiences among Indigenous communities in the American Southwest. By providing a racialized firmament for comparison that trafficked in developmental differences between "savages" and civilized people, Bourke provided the foundation for the articulation of a civilized form of settler-colonial disgust in the bodies and practices of others.

Reflecting on his observation of the practice of Indigenous North Americans delousing one another, and as part of the practice consuming the insects they find on each other's bodies, Bourke cannot help but find the experience "disagreeable." He goes on to describe the practice as "disgusting," indexing his affective difference from the people he observes, for whom the practice is noted as particularly intimate. In the last instance, Bourke attempts to reconcile the practice as medicinal, but cannot:

> The author of this work knows, from disagreeable personal experience and observation, that the Indians of North America very generally were addicted to the disgusting practice of cleaning each other's heads and putting all captured prey in their mouths. Such an office was considered a very delicate attention to be paid by a woman to her husband or lover, or from male friend to male friend, while on a campaign. No instance was noted of the use in a medical sense of these troublesome parasites.[44]

By his own reasoning, Bourke can explain this practice as a survival, but that does not absolve his experience of disgust. It is almost as if the practice as a survival is the central problem; the content of the act is one "disagreeable" element, but the whole of the practice and its affective register (as an intimate act between community members as they care for each other) places it into the realm of "disgust." Bourke's reaction points to how intimacy grows out of rejecting or unsettling disgust, a trope that will be returned to in chapter 4. Developing this intimacy depends on overcoming the unsympathetic responses that disgust engenders. Similarly, he attempts to account for how individuals and communities can come to accept as normal practices that civilized observers would find "loathsome" due to their association with particular materials and as evidence of social mores unfit for more civilized societies:

> It might perhaps be well to consider whether or not the constant use of and familiarity with human urine and ordure in houses, arts, and industries of various kinds would have a tendency to blunt the sensibilities of rude races, so that in their rites we could look for the introduction of these loathsome materials; just as we find that all those races whose women are allowed to go naked place a very slight value upon chastity.[45]

In bundling these associations between substances, bodies, and forms of comportment, Bourke moves from the use of "loathsome" materials among "rude races" to the devaluing of chastity among those same communities. Such a movement does what other colonial thinkers do in associating specific practices related to the use of particular substances with the qualities of a society as a whole. Whatever sympathies Bourke may have had for the Zuñi and other communities he worked with, there is an unfortunate way that his civilized disgust shines through, particularly in his understanding of the sympathetic relationship between the substances that people use and their character as a race, "rude" or civilized. Rejecting sympathetic interactions lays the basis for allopathic practice and works to differentiate emerging settler-colonial forms of medical expertise from Indigenous practices.

## Sympathetic Magic and Medicine's Operation

What Bourke's unilineal perspective uncovers for him is the straight line between early religious practices and latter-day medicine, which demonstrates that there is a shared association between malady and cure. This chafes against allopathic expectations that there should be an inverted relationship between disease and treatment based on an unsympathetic relation; homeopathy and other competing medical practices—including "folk" healing ways of Indigenous communities—can then be construed as backward in relation to a growing consensus that allopathic medicine represents the success of the scientific method in creating a form of medicine that is effective against disease. Yet Bourke's underlying conception of medicine as operating through sympathetic relationships is difficult to shake.[46] Because Bourke accepts religion and medicine developing together, they mutually inform each other's practice and the beliefs that surround them, both by practitioners and consumers. Moreover, in the broader social context in which they exist, expectations about the practice of medicine and religion and the institutions that support them lead to entrenchments of beliefs that, while they might be explicitly repressed, endure even when they are largely discredited. Bourke demonstrates this in his working through of categorical distinctions between religion and medicine, witchcraft and pharmacy, the first of which is irrational and the latter the product of reason. Nonetheless, the result for the use of excremental medicine was that it became associated with backwardness, witchcraft, and superstition; excremental medicine became something that stands in opposition to developing ideas of whiteness in the United States because of its association with religion and magic, backwardness and racialized difference.

Bourke's survey of the sympathetic relationship between medicine and malady leads him to focus on European alchemy as a parallel practice to the religious healing practices of nonwhite communities located in Europe's colonies. Alchemical traditions provide him with a protoscientific practice that is based in part in empirical observation and help to narrate a break between "savage" practices and the protosciences that laid the basis for civilization in the North Atlantic. That these alchemical observations are based largely on sympathetic relationships between the substance and its intended and perceived effects draws a connecting line between the alchemical and the ceremonial use of excremental medicine. The following alchemical recipe involves fermenting the urine of a preadolescent boy in horse manure and then pouring it on human feces in order to create a distilled medicinal substance. Its wide application is an index of both its perceived potency and the believed roots of many diseases in associations with impurity leading to illness. Bourke writes, glossing his historical sources:

> Then there was a "*spiritus urinre per putrefactionem.*" To make this, the urine of a boy twelve years old, who had been drinking wine, was placed in a receptacle, surrounded by horse-dung for forty days, allowed to putrefy, then decanted upon human ordure, and distilled in an alembic, etc. . . . The resulting fluid was looked upon as a great "anodyne" for all sorts of pains, and given both internally and externally, as well as in scurvy, hypochondria, cachexy, yellow and black jaundice, calculi of the kidneys and bladder, epilepsy, and mania. "Potable gold" was made from this spirit.[47]

That this surely fragrant substance could be consumed is a testament to its symbolic ability to transcend the associations the included substances individually have with dirt and disorder; it also may be that, as a bundle of materials that are objectionable into one ur-substance, the taboo related to its use is so profound as to propel the substance into an entirely different conceptual register. To that end, that it could be understood by its users as "potable gold" must be predicated on precisely this kind of alchemical transformation of something disgusting into its opposite. In that transformation, "potable gold" abides by the same logic as the Feast of Fools and its variations: through transgression, order is upheld. Moreover, some exceptional potency is derived from the excremental, alchemically transmuting waste into something seemingly beyond valuation.

Similarly, in the following, Bourke discusses at length the purported efficacy of excremental medicine in the context of European alchemy.

> Flemming remarks that those who could use urine, calculi, and things of that kind in medical practice, should not shrink from the employment of ordure as well. "And it is truly wonderful," he says, "that a

substance, the very aspect and odor of which are sufficient to induce an inevitable nausea, should be regarded not merely as a matter of curiosity and study, but held in the highest repute as a unique and most precious treasure for the preservation of health." Yet Paracelsus, and others of his school, knowing the natural repugnance to the acceptance of such medicines, prepared it under the name of "Zibethum Occidentalis," and administered it in doses of from one to two drams, given in honey or wine, to ward off attacks of fever; by others, it was employed as a plaster in cases of throat inflammation, being then called "Aureum." Others again were of the opinion, from an examination of its chemical nature, that it was fairly entitled to a place in the Materia Medica. An oil and water were distilled from it, and used in ocular sores, corrosive ulcers, and all sorts of fistulas; for affections of the scalp, for the ulcers of erysipelas, for ring-worm and tetter, and especially the pains of gout. Finally, it was believed by many to be of exceptional efficacy in the cure of the plague, being taken internally.[48]

"Inevitable nausea" confirms the disgusting nature of the substance; yet, like "potable gold," its alchemical properties transcended its symbolic associations—or inverted them to the extent that the power of "Zibethum Occidentalis" was derived from its evocation of disgust. That one might consume it to fight plague indexes the forms of desperation that motivated its use: it was not a medicine of first recourse, but something employed in life-threatening circumstances. Named for the civet cat, which produces a strong musk, Zibethum Occidentalis places the origins of the civet cat in the Occident, as opposed to its native tropics of Asia and Africa. It becomes, in its naming, white feces with the power of purification.

At its foundation, Bourke accepts that all medicine is fundamentally rooted in a set of beliefs about substances and their sympathetic powers. However far modern medicine might get from its roots, however unsympathetic it may become, it is conceptually indebted to the mimetic and metonymic relationships between substances and their relationships to human bodies. This ultimately grounds medicine in the human body itself, and the way that "awe" was inspired by the body and its emissions: "The grandest animal of all, man, could not well be omitted from the Materia Medica; every thing that pertains to either sex, either in structure or in function, must have impressed the untutored mind with a sense of awe; all excretions, solid or fluid, were invested with mystic properties, and called into requisition upon occasions of special import."[49] Taming that "awe" through the implementation of substances as medicine produced an early materia medica, a sort of primordial accumulation based in the body and its products,[50] and provided a means to tame nature through deliberate action upon it. Disgust, for Bourke, is based in the body, and so are the powers that derive from the abject. Rather than having their power based in their difference from the body, they derive their power from their "sympathetic" associations: "Medicines themselves were nothing but charms originally, in the application of which our forefathers paid less attention to pharmaceutical properties than they did to those of an occult or 'sympathetic' nature which their own ignorance attributed to them."[51] Medicine, religion, and magic, for Bourke, are inseparable, not simply because of the set of beliefs they are embedded in within a society, but because they are fundamentally tied to the human body and its byproducts. This can be a problem for categorical distinctions; it can also be a problem for conceptualizing what medicine and magic are seeking to do and the contexts of their applicable differences.

This challenge of categorical and practical distinctions between medicine and its precursors is most clearly elaborated when Bourke attempts to distinguish the differences between the effects of substances and the accepted basis of disease, here captured in his use of "known" and "obscure." Writing before the wide acceptance of the germ theory of disease and the revolutions in medicine that would occur alongside the increased use of laboratory technologies, in retrospect none of the "known" causes of disease were likely verifiable; instead, even in the late nineteenth century, many physicians and patients likely labored under the continued influence of miasma theory and environmental and constitutional conceptions of etiology.[52] He writes, attempting to make a distinction between Pharmacy/medicine and Witchcraft/magic:

> Under "Pharmacy," therefore, have been retained all remedies for the alleviation of known disorders, while under "Witchcraft" are tabulated all that were to be administered or applied for the amelioration of ailments of an obscure type, the origin of which the ignorant suf-

ferer would unhesitatingly seek in the malevolence of supernatural beings or in the machinations of human foes possessed of occult influences. Side by side with these, very properly go all such aids as were believed to insure better fortune in money-making, travelling, etc.[53]

On one side, Bourke associates "known disorders" with the efficacies of medicine to treat them, laying the foundation for a modern materia medica through the elaboration of a contemporary, scientifically grounded Pharmacy; on the other side, Witchcraft is intended to include the care for not only diseases that are "obscure" but also typically superstitious beliefs. This passage appears in a chapter on "Amulets and Talismans," where Bourke attempts to distinguish between the use of ineffectual trinkets made from human and nonhuman excrement and the ingestion of excremental medicine. At once he attends to the psychological benefits of an excremental talisman as a placebo of sorts and the seeming efficacy of the application and ingestion of excremental medicine. If both are effective, distinguishing between Pharmacy and Witchcraft casts those who employ talismans and amulets as somehow more backward than those who practice a "rational" medicine based on "known" diseases, on their etiologies and treatments.

Given the route that Bourke follows to build the relationship among medicine, religion, and magic, one might be suspect of the claim in the following that, "until the present century," it has been impossible to lose the effects of superstition in medicine; instead, what becomes clear in his invocation of nonwhite races is that the suppression of superstition is integral to producing whiteness through medicine, a fundamental repression in the making of civilization.

> Medicine, both in theory and practice, even among nations of the highest development and refinement, has not, until within the present century, cleared its skirts of the superstitious handprints of the dark ages. With tribes of a lower degree of culture it is still subordinate to the incantations and exorcisms of the "medicine man." It might not be going a step too far to assert that the science of therapeutics, pure and simple, has not yet taken form among savages; but to shorten discussion and avoid controversy, it will be assumed here that such a science does exist, but in an extremely rude and embryotic

state; and to this can be referred all examples of the introduction of urine or ordure in the materia medica, where the aid of the "medicine man" does not seem to have been invoked, as in the method employed for the eradication of dandruff by Mexicans, Eskimo, and others, the Celtiberian dentifrice, etc.[54]

While extending the possibility of a "savage" science to "rude" and "embryotic" cultures and the possibility of a primitive role such as the "medicine man" (more witch than physician), he purposefully invokes nonwhite societies as multitudinous—"Mexicans, Eskimo, and others"—against the specificity of the proto-whiteness of Celts. In the use of "savage" science and medicine men, the use of excremental medicine is effective in treating the disease complaint or maintaining health, in this case the eradication of dandruff and promotion of dental health; in both cases, excremental medicine might be taken to be used more widely, given its proven efficacy. But the association of the excremental with backwardness, here associated explicitly with race, casts this usage as superstitious and dangerous. Despite this, Bourke allows for the possibility that there are "savage" practices inside any of us, an effect of the proximity of medicine to other expert forms of knowing the world and practicing on bodies.

> Exactly where the science of medicine ended, and the science of witchcraft began, there is no means of knowing; like Astrology and Astronomy, they were twin sisters, issuing from the same womb, and travelling amicably hand in hand for many years down the trail of civilization's development; long after medicine had won for herself a proud position in the world of thought and felt compelled through shame to repudiate her less-favored comrade in public, the strictest and closest relations were maintained in the seclusion of private life.[55]

What happens in the privacy of one's own home lies beyond the power of social norms to entirely shape; instead, the superstitions associated with religion and magic and the consumption of excremental medicine might persist despite efforts to separate them from medical practice. Where they might most clearly be demonstrated as persisting are in practices around foodways, where the powers of the microbial, although not known as such, shaped foods and their consumption. In so doing, they may have acted medicinally as well. But the recognition of the microbial as such was subsumed in associations between the excremental as shit, the contamination of food, and the people who consume it.

## The Early Microbiotic and Unsympathetic Medicine

Quoting a letter from Dr. Gustav Jaeger from Stuttgart, Bourke writes:

> The neighbors of an establishment famous for its excellent bread, pastry, and similar products of luxury, complained again and again of the disgusting smells which prevailed therein and which penetrated into their dwellings. The appearance of cholera finally lent force to these complaints, and the sanitary inspectors who were sent to investigate the matter found that there was a connection between the water-closets of these dwellings and the reservoir containing the water used in the preparation of the bread. This connection was cut off at once, but the immediate result thereof was a perceptible deterioration of the quality of the bread. Chemists have evidently no difficulty in demonstrating that water impregnated with "extract of water-closet," has the peculiar property of causing dough to rise particularly fine, thereby imparting to bread the nice appearance and pleasant flavor which is the principal quality of luxurious bread.[56]

From the vantage of the early twenty-first century, it is obvious that it was the microbiota in the "extract of water-closet" that had this "luxurious" effect on the yeast and wheat that was pleasing consumers. The problem is that, in its moment and still in the present, excrement has become so associated with shit and disease, particularly in the wake of the growing understanding of its role in the cause and spread of cholera, that it cannot be food. Although there might have been a quiet desire by some of its consumers to keep manufacturing bread with "extract of water-closet," it became impossible due to the symbolic relationship between shit and contamination.

Racism's reliance on associations between kinds of people and kinds of substances necessarily barred the inclusion of racialized medicines as part of the materia medica of a burgeoning biomedicine, grounded in an unsympathic, allopathic ontology. Whatever benefits the excremental might have been understood to have at one point (whether based in magic or some early medicine), shit was becoming associated with the dirt of colonialism and emergent ideas about racial difference. Cleaning up the pollution associated with the leaky water closets also meant eradicating the microbial and its influence on human health—for good and ill.

Similarly, Bourke turns to accounts of cheese-making and the use of urine as a fermenting agent in the aging of dairy. He ascribes the origins of the practices as a superstitious ward against witches, but simultaneously recognizes that the use of urine is effective in producing food that people want to eat—and the implication is that they are willing to, despite knowing about the use of urine in this way:

> Whether or not the use of human urine to ripen cheese originated in the ancient practice of employing excrementitious matter to preserve the products of the dairy from the maleficence of witches; or, on the other hand, whether or not such an employment as an agent to defeat the efforts of the witches be traceable to the fact that stale urine was originally the active ferment to hasten the coagulation of the milk would scarcely be worth discussion.[57]

That the excremental was part of the diet of Europeans and settlers in North America is well established through Bourke's survey, whether or not consumers knew they were participating in eating the microbial. In explicit and implicit ways, the excremental had become part of everyday life for many settlers, both as an object of superstition and as the basis for medicinal, dietary, or ceremonial ritual practice. In the high colonial period that Bourke was writing in, managing the boundaries between legitimate and illegitimate uses of the excremental was increasingly bound up in ideas about civilization and race, with a strong impetus toward the elimination of the excremental, and by extension a reliable source of the microbial as well. The effect of this distancing constructs settler-colonial disgust in the other and their practices. It places disgust outside of the self and situates it as a response to other people.

For me, Bourke provides a glimpse of how human societies and human nature were being articulated in the nineteenth century. He is sympathetic to the people he is stationed with, yet he can't help but be disgusted by their practices, or at least the practices of the clowns among them. His pursuit in *Scatalogic Rites* is a rationalization of the practices that he observes: rather than take the Zuñi as fundamentally different from white settlers, he wants to be able to position them as kin in the great web of humanity. In situating their practices as shared across human societies and across time, he aims to make them kin. But doing so enrolls him in a conceptual project that racializes practices, one that reflects his sense of disgust, which moves from a substance, to a practice, to a people. That attitude also reflects the growing, dominant conception of how medicine should act and what it should be made of, which worked to preclude traditional medical practices from an emerging allopathic hegemony. This isn't Bourke's fault so much as he is representative of broader attitudes among settlers in the late nineteenth century.

The "urine dance" that Bourke witnesses is alarming to him because it transgresses a boundary that he accepted as resolute. It was doubly shocking to him because of the esteem he held for the Zuñi as, if not civilized by the standards of American settlers, then civilized by the standards of the increasingly colonized and repressed peoples of North America. Throughout his analysis, Bourke struggles to differentiate the use of excrement as medicine from the superstitious interactions people have with it, both as an object of ritual and as an everyday taboo. What is clear, however, is that the continued use of the excremental as something that is consumed is consistently associated with a prior civilizational state, and one that is increasingly associated with nonwhite, colonized not colonizing, societies. In this way, the excremental becomes something to be governed in much the same ways that colonized communities need to be governed. By extension, the interactions between people and the things they consume, whether medicine or food, become governed too. Bourke uses terms like "restrict" to associate the use of the excremental with "rude races" and implies that a break has been made among white settler-colonial societies from the superstitious and dangerous ways of earlier phases of civilization.

As a token of a way of thinking, Bourke is exemplary. He narrates the growing consensus—likely largely unspoken but often implied—about the need to clean up settler-colonial societies, and by extension to purify its medicines of their premodern pasts. While not instrumental in this shift, Burke indexes a broader trend in the United States and elsewhere away from the microbial in its form as excremental, with the articulation of allopathic medicine making a fundamental break from its precursors and competitors, homeopathy foremost among them. It is attitudes like Bourke's that lay the foundation for what was to come in the early twentieth century, as John Harvey Kellogg and his contemporaries elaborated the basis of the Standard American Diet and its basis in purity and regularity based in racial ideology.

# Threshold 1
## POROUS BODIES

IS ALEXIS ST. MARTIN the person who made me what I am today? I'm not sure when I first learned about St. Martin, but in terms of childhood lessons, it was an indelible one. St. Martin was working for a fur trading company in 1822 in my home state of Michigan when he was accidentally shot in the chest with a musket. Fired from just a meter away, the duck shot that pierced his abdomen blew apart a few of his ribs and punctured his stomach. At the fort where he was working, there was a staff surgeon, William Beaumont, who rushed to St. Martin's aid. Beaumont was able to stuff St. Martin's lower lung back into his chest, remove fragments of bone and duck shot, and apply bandages to St. Martin to stop the bleeding and protect the wound. As was the state of the medical arts of the time, Beaumont bled St. Martin to stabilize his condition. St. Martin was wracked with an infection over the coming days, and yet he survived. Was the wound also a vehicle for microbial colonization, making him "unusually plethoric and robust"?[1] Take, for instance, this aside from Beaumont's account of St. Martin's life: In 1832, "he was in the midst of the cholera epidemic . . . and withstood its ravages with impunity, while hundreds around him fell sacrifices to its fatal influence."[2] Might that "impunity" have been a microbially aided capacity provided by his wound? Beaumont goes on to write that St. Martin had "suffered much less predisposition to disease than is common to men of his age and circumstances in life."[3] It may be St. Martin's especially porous body that extended his life and protected him from illness.

Some hiccup of physiology resulted in St. Martin's stomach creating a fistula with his epidermis. This fistula, as Beaumont would describe it, created a kind of "anus," an opening into St. Martin's body. If it was an anus, it was unlike any other. It was a hole large enough to put one's finger into and, as Beaumont would soon learn, serve as the source for a series of experiments on human digestion. Beaumont describes it as a "perforation . . . about two and a half inches in circumference, and the food and drinks constantly exuded, unless prevented by a tent, compress and bandage."[4] Beaumont's experiments transfixed me as a child, as I wondered what it was like to dangle a piece of food into an open wound, what it was like to have food dangled into one's body, and how a person could live with a perpetual additional orifice.

Over the next decade, St. Martin and Beaumont embarked on an ambivalent relationship. St. Martin was financially dependent on Beaumont, who employed him as a servant and general laborer; and Beaumont was dependent on St. Martin, as his reputation as an experimentalist and physician was slowly growing as a result of his access to St. Martin, and particularly St. Martin's digestive processes. Over their decade together, Beaumont reports having conducted some two hundred experiments. Many of them involved Beaumont extracting gastric juices from St. Martin's body or tying a piece of food to a string and dangling it into St. Martin's stomach, as the wound never closed. Instead, St. Martin's body somehow created a sort of interior valve that could be pushed aside to permit Beaumont his desired access.[5] Over time, Beaumont came to understand how digestion worked, from the composition of gastric juices to the comparative rates of different kinds of food being broken down for metabolization. He also came to learn how a relationship built on indebtedness and exploitation soured whatever friendship he might have had with St. Martin, who, at least twice that Beaumont records, ran away to his native Canada until he was destitute enough to need to return to Beaumont. Eventually, though, St. Martin was able to extricate himself from the relationship with Beaumont and lived out the rest of his life without the burden of being treated as an experimental subject. Because of expressed interest on the part of the U.S. military in preserving his stomach as a medical curiosity, his family left his body to rot in their home until it was in a state too decomposed to preserve before reporting his death. After the funeral, they interred St. Martin under eight feet of earth, hoping to dissipate the curiosities around his body and its opening into the body's processes.

How could his family have known that St. Martin would become a medical curiosity that was recurrently written about over the next two centuries? How could they know the strange pride my home state would find in St. Martin, so much that I would learn about St. Martin in elementary school? How could they know that Beaumont's influence would be so profound that the local network of hospitals my father would work for would be named after him, nearly a hundred years after his death? How could they know the spell St. Martin's "anus" would cast on me as a child, so powerful that I would return to it again and again, curious about his experience of the world?

Now I return to St. Martin because he literalizes the porous body that contemporary conceptions of the microbial allow. Beaumont was interested in the molar, those pieces of food that were obvious objects that could be put into St. Martin's body through his aperture; I am interested in the molecular, those largely imperceptible creatures that permeate the body and make digestion possible. Beaumont was able to discern the chemical process involved and was able to confirm that human bodies create hydrochloric acid to break down food into its molecular parts. But what he was unable to perceive, and what might have seemed to be absolutely premodern superstition, was the activity of microbial actors working away at the fraying molecular components of food. He also likely couldn't imagine how St. Martin's open body was a vehicle for microbes to pass in and out of it; St. Martin was an even stranger experiment than Beaumont could know. Maybe St. Martin's long life, as he lived into his seventies, was the result of this steady flow of microbial agents, making him the first truly microbial man. St. Martin offers an early figuration of the body as landscape, where the inside of the body and its exterior bleed together into one terrain, eased through St. Martin's second "anus." That opening, which mixes body and environment, also blurs the distinctions between humans and their natural world, which often rests on the spurious distinction between civilization and nature.

Bodies tend to be conceptualized as whole, discrete objects that are permeable only in specific ways, say through an orifice or wound. This is the production of the body as a molar object, which Gilles Deleuze and Félix Guattari juxtapose to the body as a molecular process.[6] Their attention to the molecular provides them with a way to conceptualize the body as something that is always in a process of becoming. Although their examples are largely metaphoric, such a conception of bodies provides a model for how molecular processes—from microbial agents to pharmaceuticals, from nutrients to toxins—shape our bodies in processual ways that make them different over time. The body as a molecular process is also the body as a landscape, one open to and coterminous with its environment in supple ways. In this respect, St. Martin's body is different in degree rather than in kind: he is explicitly open to his environment, his "anus" providing an aperture that microbes can traffic through, even if they are imperceptible and unknown to him. Similarly, we are all affected by unknown and imperceptible agents, but our current microbial turn seeks to describe these relationships and unsettle dominant conceptions of the molar body as separate from nature in fundamental ways.

Nature and civilization are often pitted against each other for the purpose of making claims about the purity of one over the other. Throughout American history, nature has been taken to exist prior to the adulterations that human activity introduces, like culture, society, civilization, development, or modernity, all of which inaugurate a break from nature, that state of prelapsarian being in which humans were undifferentiated from the natural milieu they were constituted through.[7] It is a tired story that gets told again and again, often to demonstrate the superiority of one group over another, which may come in the form of either being closer to nature or being further removed from it. On one side are "noble savages" and "virgin land," and on the other, developed, technocratic, civilized states, the latter represented in American settlers and the former by Indigenous inhabitants. Food and medicine get caught in these projects as well, from old anthropological concerns with the advent of fire, which inaugurated a nutritional and cognitive rupture from our evolutionary past,[8] to structuralist concerns about the "raw" and the "cooked," which index the relative associations between qualities ascribed to everyday objects, like the food we eat.[9] Similarly, medicine has, from the late nineteenth century onward, been split into civilized, industrially produced pharmaceuticals and evidence-based interventions, on the one hand, and the natural, alternative, non-Western medicines available without prescriptions in health food stores and the relatively unregulated complementary medical traditions that have circulated as consumer goods and practices, on the other.[10] Wherever the distinction between nature and civilization appears, and whatever form it takes, it draws a line between one person or community and another; drawing that distinction is an operation of power that can serve to denigrate people and practices or reclaim them as vital traditions.[11]

If John Bourke and others of his generation and their successors sought to use proximity to nature as a means to denigrate and control communities, associating particular people and their rituals with being "backward" and uncivilized through their association with the excremental, they also produced the foundations for the deployment of a proximity to nature as the basis for critique of racist, civilizing projects. This has been most apparent, recently, in returns and appreciations of nonwhite foodways. If one of the effects that people like John Harvey Kellogg and Adelle Davis had (discussed in the following two chapters) was the construction of a Standard American Diet that reflected the values of a dominant, white society in the United States[12]—even if it changed over time and was influenced by industrial investments and government subsidies— they also helped to provide the grounds on which counterdiscourses of diet and food could be developed. In the United States, this has recently flourished in scholarship about Black and Indigenous foodways, as well as a surge in related popular cookbooks.[13] Scholars and cooks have sought to counteract a century or more of bigoted dietary thinking that has diminished the social and nutritional vitality of once-marginalized eating practices,[14] and in doing so, they have done critical work in connecting historical conditions of deprivation to the canny survival strategies of individuals and communities that have created the basis for long-standing culinary and medical practices.[15] The deprivation that many communities faced over the course of the long colonial efforts of white settlers in North America led to forms of innovation that created discoveries in edibility and curative properties that, when protected, can serve as the basis for intellectual property and long-standing community practices.

One of the sites of the power of these discourses around a return to nature lies in the dirt that is associated with the natural world and the way that "dirty" food and medicine disrupts whiteness and its claims to purity. Fermented foods are one of these substances. At their core, they are rotten, having become contaminated by microbes.[16] But, over time and through experimentation, humans have come to relish certain fermented foods despite their apparent spoiled nature; they have come to accept that the "dirt" is part of the pleasure in consuming the food.[17] This echoes one of the central problems in excremental medicine, as described by Bourke. The very idea of consuming "dirt" disrupts purity and becomes associated with risks, both to the individual body and to the body politic as a composite of a bodies and the substances they consume. If there is a steady lesson provided by the small current of scholars interested in excrement and its powers, it is this: shit, as both substance and symbol, strikes at the heart of civilization and its claims to purification.[18] Daily, human waste is created and in need of being flushed away; this creates the need for infrastructures of disappearance that first hide and then either remake waste into something useful like compost or fertilizer or return it to nature. But the challenge is that, even excrement is a product of civilization, itself a byproduct of the foods we eat, the consumer markets that make it available and desirable, and the agricultural systems that produce that food and rely on the processing of human waste to make nutritional foods. Food and excrement are intrinsically linked, both in our physiological processes and in how they work and rework nature and civilization in our everyday experiences.

Awareness of this integral relationship between civilization and waste is not a way out of the constant debates about and consumerist repurposing of nature and its opposites. There is no purity to be found in an uncontaminated nature that was never really there, nor in the industrially produced cleanliness that is a byproduct of a sanitized society. Instead, the important thing is the project itself, how nature is constantly worked and reworked in new ways that thereby create emergent opportunities for encounters with the wild, the untamed, and the unsettled. This can lead to strange bedfellows, as in the case of bioprospecting medicines through partnerships between field scientists, Indigenous communities, and multinational pharmaceutical conglomerates.[19] It can also lead to the revitalization of transnational communities through a shared interest in historical foodways that have served as oppositional sites for the articulation of individual and group identities. There are dangers, such as Indigenous communities being robbed of their intellectual property and a politics of authenticity creating marginalized communities within already marginalized communities, but the play of and with nature is a critical tool is disrupting racist claims to civilization and the exclusions such claims make possible.

The human body as a molar object is a success of unsympathetic medicine. Another version of St. Martin and Beaumont's relationship and St. Martin as an experimental subject might have trundled down a path that attempted to reconcile St. Martin's increased porousness with his recovery, his ongoing well-being, and his molecular nature. Did the wound that further opened his body to the environment, leading to an imperceptible and unknowable stream of microbial agents, also lead to his recovery? Such a conception of the body as molecular, as a landscape, erodes the distinction between nature and civilization, which depends on the division between bodies and the environments they inhabit. The Enlightenment project of civilization was predicated on the understanding that humans, unlike other animals, were unique in their ability to transcend the determinants of their surroundings. Civilization created a barrier between humans and their environments, extricating them from nature and rendering their bodies discrete, knowable, molar objects. As objects, they are machines, and their functioning is chemical, which Beaumont was able to elucidate. But in so doing, he described only part of what was occurring.

It might seem unfair, and unsympathetic, to read Beaumont as incapable of or uninterested in conceptualizing the body differently. But the molar body as machine or body as object was the result of an ongoing process in scientific thought that worked against dominant ways of conceptualizing the body as influenced by its environment, nowhere better described than in miasmatic theory, which accepted that the body was susceptible to the atmospheres it moved through or that moved through it. Strong smells were often indicative of miasmatic spaces, making charnel houses and garbage piles and open sewers all suspect as sites for disease—which they may have been, but not in the way that then-contemporary science described the process. Microscopy and the other technologies that would permit sensing the microbial world were still decades away from being refined, so it is not so much that Beaumont could (literally) have seen differently, as it is that St. Martin's accident offered an opportunity to keep alive a different way of conceptualizing the body and its environmental interactions. Instead, Beaumont constructed St. Martin's body as separate from the natural influences that might have affected it.

In this way, Beaumont participated in the development of a particularly unsympathetic medicine, which was reflected in his relationship with St. Martin. If I was drawn to St. Martin's story as a child because of its body horror (and in many ways, I still am), now the unsympathetic relationship that Beaumont developed with St. Martin is equally revealing of the currents in the development of American medicine in the nineteenth century. Their relationship reflects the growing conception of the body as separate and separable from its environment, a processual understanding that Beaumont aided in developing through his treatment of St. Martin as a machine to be experimented with. And it's in Beaumont's callousness that the body horror blooms into something unsympathetic: putting his finger into St. Martin's body through his fistula-anus, dangling food in his stomach, coercing St. Martin into a research relationship predicated on St. Martin's economic precarity and in the service of Beaumont's standing in American medicine as an elite profession. St. Martin was the perfect subject for such unsympathetic treatment, existing as he did on the frontiers of American settler colonialism along the borderlands of the United States and Canada. As a voyageur, St. Martin existed through his labor in the fissure between nature and civilization, serving as an interface between Indigenous and settler communities, aiding in the harvesting of the fauna of the frontiers of American expansionism for the benefit of markets in urbanizing metropoles on the Eastern Seaboard. He was precarious, and that precarity led him to depend on Beaumont. Like Bourke, Beaumont provided a view into another world, and while they might seem to be worlds apart from the vantage of the twenty-first century, at the time they were both views onto nature divorced from civilization. To secure that split between the natural world and the civilizations that humans can cultivate, Beaumont acted on St. Martin in an unsympathetic way that worked to reify nature as objectifiable, as something that interacts with our bodies, but which must be regulated in its contact. From such a conception of the body, diet becomes an everyday project that provides a way to act on the body and its exposures.

# 2 The Rise of the American Diet
## THE SAVAGE WITHIN AND THE REGULATION OF WHITENESS

The Colon Not a Sewer: What natural reason can be shown that food that enters the body clean, sweet and sterile should leave the body in a state horribly loathsome with corruption?

—John Harvey Kellogg, *Dr. Kellogg's Lectures on Practical Health Topics*

WILLIAM AND JOHN HARVEY KELLOGG made the modern American breakfast. Coming out of the nineteenth century, with a background in the vegetarianism of Seventh Day Adventism, the Kellogg brothers argued that the meat-heavy diet that white Americans inherited from their European ancestors, filled with salted meats and starchy carbohydrates, like potatoes, was both individually unhealthy and leading to "race degeneracy," a slow form of unwitting eugenics that white Americans were indulging in despite their best individual and national interests. The Kellogg-led American breakfast that embraced toasted grains, of which corn flakes was the paradigmatic form, sought to purify Americans from within. Cereal offered a return to nature, a means to counteract the effects of a corrupting settler-colonial life, where the increased sedentariness, removal from natural settings, and rise of processed foods threatened to erode the health of Americans. Taken for granted as it is, the invention of modern breakfast cereals was an enormous culinary achievement, having taken William years of experimentation to achieve:[1] cooked grains, dried, and packaged for mass consumption made breakfast require a fraction of the time it did previously, shaping the possibilities of American everyday life in new ways by creating surplus time to invest elsewhere.

The Kelloggs worked in partnership for part of their careers, but eventually existed in an acrimonious relationship, with William managing the burgeoning food industry and John Harvey leading the Battle Creek Sanitorium. John was a leading public intellectual in the late nineteenth and early twentieth centuries, publishing both popular and scholarly books, while William operated largely behind the scenes, managing the business of growing the Kellogg brand. John was immediately recognizable for many Americans; he was the face of a growing discourse around "wellness" that was central to the practice of the Battle Creek Sanitorium, which focused on the regularity of diet, exercise, and sleep. The cereals were central to this project and worked synergistically with John's public persona, but by the end of his life, his sanitorium had become bankrupt and his nineteenth-century views of allopathic medicine had become outdated, as many were based on crude science and preindustrial medicine. Meanwhile, Kellogg's cereal had become a multinational, multimillion-dollar business. Yet, if the Kellogg brothers have indelibly shaped the American diet in obvious ways, the subtle influence of John's thinking more often goes unnoticed and unremarked.

In this chapter, I focus on how John Harvey Kellogg (hereafter just "Kellogg") constituted American whiteness through the development of a set of interlocking ideas about regularity, taste, and race. Throughout his work, regularity is a central concept that he employs to discuss physiological processes, the structure of everyday life, and the interactions between individuals and their environments. This regularity is both diagnostic and therapeutic: if something is wrong with a body, it will be evident in its irregularity and can be addressed by restoring regularity through proper dieting and exercise. The challenge Kellogg identifies is that the American palate has led Americans astray, as they have wandered in their diets away from the needs associated with "physiological eating." Americans have come to eat not according to their body's needs, but according to their desires. This has led to digestive issues, and an erosion of health more generally. For Kellogg, this is a sign of "race degeneracy," a corruption associated with civilization that is leading to the fall of white Americans. Whiteness, for Kellogg, is inextricable from its associations with a particular regularity based on its dietary purity and relationship to American everyday life as it became structured by early twentieth century capitalism, encapsulated in work and school days.

Writing about Kellogg is an exercise in both national and local history. As a Michigander, Kellogg has been a part of my personal history, both because of the proximity of the Battle Creek Sanitarium to where I grew up and because of his status as a celebrity in Michigan history. Like St. Martin and Beaumont, Kellogg is a figure who is well represented in histories of Michigan and its role in the United States, and because of the ubiquity of Kellogg's cereals—despite their actual association with his brother—Kellogg and his work are woven into American everyday life to the degree that assumptions about whole-grain-based breakfasts are commonsense elements in American diets. But this ubiquity belies the depth and impact of his work, which was widely read and circulated in public discourse. Kellogg was constantly promoting his work, and his purchase in American attitudes toward the body and dietary practices cannot be overstated, in no small part because his attitudes reflected dominant norms. Some of those ideas now feel quite dated, but I have found that it is not those that are obviously outdated, such as his ideas about putrefaction, that are the hardest to confront, but the ones that have become embedded in American lifeways, such as his conception of "regularity" and its basis in dietary practices. This diet-based regularity might be cast as "objective," yet this objective status was earned through his dedicated self-promotion and the ways that assumptions about diet and regularity have worked their way into American common sense about bodies and their processes. Like many Americans, I largely accept these tenets of Kellogg's, but that acceptance exists in tension with their troubling history.

Here, I focus first on Kellogg's conception of human physiology and its rhythmic regularity. From this basis in the body, I turn toward his understanding of diet and how it influences and reflects rhythms in diet's associations with regularity and the need for individual regulation through consumption. I then turn to the role that race plays in his thinking, which serves both as a foil for whiteness, in his invocation of "noble savages" and their relation to nature, and as what dangers lie ahead for white Americans if they continue to eat poorly. In the end, I engage with Kellogg's work on putrefaction and autointoxication as his most sustained foray into the dangers of the microbial and its contact with the human body. Taken together, Kellogg's conception of regularity lays the basis for whiteness and the dangers associated with straying from nature through an embrace of civilization. Like the natural-foods advocates that would follow him, his solution for this lapse was a reintroduction of proximity to nature through diet, which becomes apparent in bodily regularities. Such an attention to regularity makes the dangers associated with corruption a daily risk to navigate, but it also produces whiteness not as a status associated solely with phenotype, but a capacity captured in the possibilities of self-cultivation through diet and wellness.

I read Kellogg's work in an idiosyncratic fashion. I focus on four of his many books, *The Stomach: Its Disorders and How to Cure Them* (1896), *The Living Temple* (1903), *Dr. Kellogg's Lectures on Practical Health Topics* (1913), and *Colon Hygiene* (1915), and read them against each other. As texts, they range from public-facing self-help books, to science-based cookbooks, to physiology textbooks. Throughout, Kellogg comes back to the same set of concerns repeatedly: autointoxication, putrefaction, vegetarianism, "savages," and regulation. In so doing, the set of ideas that animate him are mobilized in different contexts for different audiences. That said, as ideas, they contain a stable set of relations that he employs repeatedly to make his points, each rooted in his conceptions of race, degeneracy, and humanity's relationship with nature and the corrupting influences of civilization. Historians are often interested in how thought develops, how it matures over time; Kellogg, however, did not mature so much as ripen. His interests remained the same, but the language he employed to make his points became richer and steeped in his sense of moral order, which found its footing in resistance to the corrupting influences of "pleasure." As a thinker, Kellogg catalyzed early-twentieth-century ideas about the body, diet, and "wellness" in his conception of "regularity" and its basis in human nature, reflected in our bodily processes, and ideally in the organization of society itself. In this way, Kellogg was scalar in his conception of life and its ordering: from the individual to the societal, order could be achieved and maintained through the regulation of what people ate and when and how they ate it and evacuated it.

Throughout his work, Kellogg is interested in the balance between "cultivation"—and its aspirational aims at becoming the right kind of civilized subject—and the "savage" impulses that lie within each of us. That inner savage is returned to repeatedly throughout his work, both in metaphorical terms and in his use of examples of Indigenous communities around the world. Like John Bourke and other thinkers before him, Kellogg accepted a linear developmental trajectory to social organization and human behavior, positing that "savages" existed at some prior developmental phase and that they could ascend to a more civilized position through careful cultivation. The ascriptions of backwardness that exist throughout Kellogg's use of these examples reflect his racist leanings, as he situates white people at the forefront of civilization. The paradox for Kellogg is that the civilization that white people have wedded themselves to is also steadily distancing them too far from a pure experience of nature, and this distancing from natural appetites and tastes is leading to "race degeneracy." The critical practice for Kellogg, then, is to cultivate one's tastes to calibrate between the nature-attuned savage within and external corrupting influences without; this requires self-regulation that an individual can embark on as a form of self-care, and can also require interventions to restore a person to wellness through intensive medical attention steeped in an attention to human nature.

## Physiological Regularity and Self-Regulation

Kellogg roots his understanding of regularity in the observable physiological processes of the body, situating the regular intake of food, its movement through the alimentary canal, and defecation as the basis for normal human functioning. It is exquisite in its simplicity, focused as it is on the everyday functions of the human body and their rhythms plotted on a diurnal day of activity and a night of sleep. In this way, he joins an understanding of the internal functioning of the body and its natural physiological processes with an awareness of the social context in which this functioning occurs. If left to its own devices and with an appropriate diet, the human body should maintain its digestive rhythm; the problem that arises in the context of modern society is that the "appetites" become unaligned with actual physiological need. "Physiological eating," for Kellogg, is eating aligned with the body's needs; any other form of eating threatens to deteriorate the body from within.

Kellogg constitutes the body and its processes in their natural state by focusing on how food moves through the body, from mouth to anus, transforming from food to excrement. Along the way, the body acts on food to move it from one state to the next, from one organ to the next. In its most basic form, he describes digestion in this way: "The food is moved along the alimentary canal, from the stomach downward, by successive contractions of the muscular walls of the intestines, known as peristaltic movements, which occur with great regularity during digestion."[2] While based in the observation of bodies and their processes, Kellogg uses "regularity" to describe the process, allowing him to connect what is happening inside the body with what is happening socially. Similarly, in the following, he invokes "regulation" as a natural process that the body undergoes, when healthy and operating normally, that allows him to consider how acts of control regarding what comes into and leaves the body might abide by an analogous process. In discussing "regulation" and its basis in human physiological functioning, he writes:

> [The] vital processes of the body have two quite independent sources of regulation—the nerve centers, on the one hand, which send out exciting and controlling nerves, and, on the other hand, internal secretions which act in relation to such great functions as muscular activity. The action of every muscle, of every gland, probably of every cell, is controlled by these remarkable and subtle substances.[3]

Grounded in the body, "regulation" serves as a mechanism to shape its interactions with the substances that it encounters, particularly as food. Characterized as "subtle," regulation serves as a means to control the body from within, and through "cultivation," from without.

In the following, Kellogg describes how the regular intake of food throughout the day results in a bowel movement at "a stated hour," a strict form of regularity. He contrasts this regular movement to "irregular" behaviors that result in constipation, a "natural" symptom that results from poor self-regulation.

> By this increased activity of the alimentary canal the fecal matters resting in the upper portion of the colon are moved downward into the rectum, thereby provoking a desire for evacuation of the bowels.

By this means, the activities set up by each meal move the contents of the intestine to their appropriate station, resulting, in healthy persons, in the discharge of the alimentary residue from the body at a stated hour each day. If a meal is omitted, or if meals are taken at irregular hours, this rhythmical action is broken up, and constipation is the natural result.[4]

"Nature" is critical for Kellogg, and he accepts that the challenge facing many modern humans is civilization, which has removed us from our natural rhythms. If left to the rhythms of nature, and in a prelapsarian state where humans and nature are inseparable—as reflected in the following through his invocation of "primitive peoples" and nonhuman primates—Kellogg understands that bowel movements would be a much more frequent occurrence as a result of a more natural diet and rhythmic structure of everyday life based in a precivilized organization of society and individual lifeways. Characterizing civilization as the problem and "abnormal habits" as the result, he writes

> The practice of moving the bowels once a day, or even less frequently is peculiar to civilized people and is a result of the sedentary life and other abnormal habits which prevail in civilization. The writer has made very thorough-going inquiry among medical missionaries and others who are acquainted with the habits of primitive peoples, and finds that the universal practice among really primitive tribes is to move the bowels three or four times a day. By inquiry at the London Zoological Gardens we learned that this habit is likewise true of the large apes. The keeper in charge of these animals assured us that the gorilla, chimpanzee and the orangutan move their bowels regularly four times a day.[5]

It is critical here that Kellogg associates "primitive peoples" and gorillas, chimpanzees, and orangutans. While race is unmarked in his use of "primitive peoples," his use of "medical missionaries" points toward his assumption that these "primitive peoples" are his contemporaries, outside the reach of contemporary "civilization." Race is implied, and his racism is of the sort that ascribes a more "natural" status to those who have yet to feel the ravages of modern civilization; Americans have corrupted themselves through modern life, and only attention to the "regular" rhythms of the body and nature can restore Americans to full health.

From its basis in physiological activity, rhythm is concretized by Kellogg in the "regular" structure of everyday life, reflected in schedules of work and school and the management of mealtimes in support of these institutionalized elements. The problem for Kellogg is that these institutionalized forms of organization chafe against our body's "natural" rhythms. As he describes it, rhythm can be produced through sleeping and eating at "stated intervals," a form of regular organization that is reflected in the bowel movements in "normal" individuals.

> There are two factors which are chiefly active in producing bowel movements in normal individuals. The first is the practice of taking food only at stated intervals, regular meal hours. The second is regularity in the hours of sleep and morning rising. The omission of a meal, or a change in the hours of meals or of sleep will at once change or destroy the rhythm of bowel movements.[6]

Through the use of "stated intervals" in the production of rhythm, "regularity" can be "cultivated," as Kellogg captures in the following: "Regularity of bowel movement is of the utmost importance. It is a function which should be assiduously cultivated."[7] That "assiduously cultivated" habit of regular bowel movements depends on aligning the body's needs with the organization of society, especially when civilization has created a disruption to the body's natural proclivities. When these habits fail, disorder prevails.

Bowel movements are how one knows that the rhythms of a body are intact, providing observers with a reliable diagnostic mechanism. Bowel movements are also how an inner disorder becomes embodied in material evidence. What constitutes a bowel movement and the consistency and smell of it serve as a means to understand what is happening inside of a body, providing a use for the waste the body emits. "The bowels should move thoroughly at least once a day, most naturally soon after breakfast. Two daily movements are better, soon after each of the principal meals. Putrid, foul-smelling stools are an indication of intestinal autointoxication, and are due to an excess of protein in the form of meat, eggs, or possibly milk. Such a condition always breeds disease."[8] In cases where an individual is diagnosed with a medical condition, the regulation of one's bowel movements becomes of paramount concern, serving as a means to heal them through diet and an imposition of rhythm. For Kellogg, it is through careful self-regulation that disorder can be overcome, as he makes clear in the following discussion of neurasthenia, in which the banning of "stimulants of any kind" is critical in restoring a body's rhythm: "The neurasthenic must eat carefully and take no stimulants of any kind. And—a matter of very grave importance in this connection—he must so regulate the bowel movements as to take care of the waste materials which have accumulated. This does not mean once a day, but three times a day."[9] Restoring a natural rhythm of "three times a day" is an effort to return an individual to a precivilized state like those apes in the zoo, implicitly tying the experience of neurasthenia to the effects of the modern everyday life of being civilized.

Similarly, not having bowel movements indicates a problem of the bodily interior, and for Kellogg, constipation is a systemic problem that can lead to "auto-intoxication," or the corruption of the body through the rotting of materials in the alimentary tract. In a concise statement of his overarching conception of human health and its relationship to nature, Kellogg writes:

> Modern medical research has demonstrated that most diseases from which human beings suffer, chronic as well as acute, are due to infection of the alimentary canal by poison-forming germs. Many scores of such germs are known. The poisons are absorbed, and give rise to a great variety of distressing maladies and symptoms. Unnatural foods and unwholesome habits of life encourage infection of the intestine by introducing poison-forming bacteria and promoting their growth. Natural food and natural habits of life combat these disease-producing infections. Hence the "simple life" is an anti-toxic life.[10]

The absence of bowel movements is the "worst" possible problem an individual can face. A reliance on nature can ensure that this is avoided, however, producing a rhythm both in eating and in bowel movements. "Constipation is the worst evil that afflicts humanity, the most dangerous of all forms of intoxication the body knows. We might, indeed, call constipation a veritable Pandora's box of mischiefs, for malignant germs, scores of varieties of them, thrive there, each kind producing its particular poison, and making possible a great variety of symptoms of chronic intestinal activity."[11] That constipation is the "worst evil that afflicts humanity" is surely hyperbolic, but when one understands that constipation is the effect of civilization and the imposition of an unnatural rhythm on the human body, it becomes clear that the problem constipation indexes is a disruption of the relationship with nature that only a "cultivated" set of habits can restore.

Rather than accept that the content, frequency, and purpose of meals have developed incidentally and separate from each other, Kellogg argues that the very structure of how Americans eat is based on the continued degradation in the content of a meal: "The modern frequency of meals is the outgrowth of the gradual losing sight of the true purpose of the eating of food, the gratification of the palate being too much considered, instead of the nourishment of the body."[12] He goes on to discuss how human eating is necessarily flexible and can be modified within reason without negative effects: "[That] the system can be well nourished on two meals a day is beyond controversy, seeing that not only did our vigorous forefathers, many centuries ago, require no more, but that thousands of persons in modern times have adopted the same custom without injury, and with most decided benefit to themselves."[13] The "true purpose" of eating food, for Kellogg, is to satisfy one's physiological needs through "nourishment." In this respect, timing is secondary to content, yet they inform each other through their spatiotemporal placement: if a person eats two meals each day, what those meals consist of is based on the time of day in which they occur and their social context. Their timing affects the alimentary processes they cue. So, while a person may eat two meals per day, the effects might still be decreased peristaltic activity, potentially leading to constipation.

Critically, nature and "cultivation" are at odds with one another in the context of modern civilization, requiring individuals to realign their bodily rhythms through careful engagement with their habitual behaviors. In the following, he describes the blight of constipation as "nearly universal," which results in the false belief that one bowel movement per day is something to be "proud" of, as if that were normal. Instead, he insists that "normal" bowel movement is based in a rhythm that is based in uncontaminated nature. In this way, he moves between the basic physiological functioning of the body and society, tying the operation of the former to the structure of the latter.

> The act of taking foods stimulates peristaltic activity and it is more than probable that if from the start an individual adhered closely to the proper diet eaten in a proper manner, and took care to attend promptly to the call of Nature, the normal intestinal rhythm would be maintained. These conditions, however, rarely exist, and in consequence constipation is so nearly universal that the average individual feels himself the proud possessor of a normal colon if his bowels move once in twenty-four hours, whereas the savage declares himself to be "horribly constipated" when his bowels move but once a day. Normal bowel rhythm unquestionably demands at least three evacuations daily.[14]

In his explicit comparison between civilized, constipated people and "savages," Kellogg aligns savages with nature and civilized people with a form of alienation from their basic physiological processes that results in a false consciousness about nature in which a single daily bowel movement is sufficient to clear the body of its wastes. This bowel movement ideology structures the experience of everyday life, situating the timing and frequency of physiological functions alongside other social obligations, like work and school time. In the following, he makes the role of "habit" plain, arguing in no uncertain terms that the problem that people face in the contemporary world is one imposed through "business," meaning American capitalism and its institutionalized schedules that impinge on nature's rhythms. He aligns meal times with the "sacred," arguing that there is nothing more important than a regularity of the body that is constituted through the regularity of society and its spatiotemporal order based in an unwavering natural order.

> The human system seems to form habits, and to be in a great degree dependent upon the performance of its functions in accordance with the habits formed. In respect to digestion this is especially observable. If a meal is taken at a regular hour, the stomach becomes accustomed to receiving food at that hour, and is prepared for it. If meals are eaten

irregularly, the stomach is taken by surprise, so to speak, and is never in a proper state of readiness for the prompt and perfect performance of its work. The habit which many professional and business men have of allowing their business to intrude upon their meal hours, frequently either wholly depriving them of a meal or obliging them to take it an hour or two later than the usual time, ultimately undermines the best digestion. The hour for meals should be considered a sacred one, not to be intruded upon except under some unusual circumstance. Eating is a matter of too momentous importance to be interrupted or delayed by matters of ordinary business or convenience.[15]

Because eating is the way that the exterior gets into the body and sets off the series of physiological responses that result in a bowel movement, its regularity is vital. For Kellogg, when an individual—or a whole society—becomes unmoored from nature through the cultivation of a set of habits that is based on an unnatural imposition, as in the case of "business," they instantiate a regime of habits that works against a human body's physiological needs. Two regimes of habit emerge, one tied to nature and its cues associated with the "normal" functioning of the body and another associated with the rhythms of civilization. In this case, civilization and "business" are isomorphic with each other, casting Kellogg's contemporary United States as one removed from nature through its commitment to a particularly alienating form of capitalism. This relation is managed through the production of an American "appetite" that substitutes "pleasure" for physiological need. In a further distancing between the individual and society, this leads to "race degeneracy." What is at stake in any individual meal is not only an individual's well-being, but potentially society as a whole. Critically, "taste" arbitrates individual desires with societal needs, and cultivating the right taste upholds individual health and the well-being of society at large.

## Habit, Taste, and the Making of the American Diet

For Kellogg, taste, when it is aligned with nature, serves to regulate the body. As he writes, taste serves as a mechanism to inform a body as to whether or not a food is needed and when a body has consumed enough of it. One of the problems facing civilized eaters is that their appetites have been "perverted" through the overuse of additives, like salt, and the masking of natural taste through the use of condiments as a form of adulterating nature. Kellogg accepts that this has been a progressive transformation over human history and that his contemporaries in the United States and western Europe are the most susceptible to overeating and wrong eating as a result of their divorce from nature. Human bodies, he suggests, know what they need and act accordingly; but civilization has interrupted these natural impulses and the body's ability to recognize what will sustain it without harm, in the form of constipation and more systemic ailments.

> While food is in the mouth it is not only chewed but tasted. The recognition of the gustatory properties of food by the nerves of taste, through reflex centers in the brain, prepares the stomach, pancreas, liver and other digestive organs for the work which they are to do. Tasting the food also in some mysterious way regulates the process of nutrition by cutting off the appetite for one food principle after another as the body has received a sufficiency of each particular item.[16]

"Taste" and "regulation" work together here, serving as the basis for self-regulation, as if the body knows how to control its intake in a natural setting. That regulation is first and foremost in the body and secondarily in society is a function of Kellogg's conception of primordial human nature. If one trusts one's body, it will fulfill its needs, but in the context of modern civilization, our tastes have been perverted in ways that lead to eating the wrong things and in ways that prove disastrous for our individual health and reflect a disjuncture between civilization and nature. The problem, as Kellogg understands it, is that Americans have been swayed by the pursuit of the "pleasures" of eating. He writes elsewhere: "The so-called pleasures of the table are usually illicit enjoyments resulting from the indulgence of artificial tastes and depraved appetites from which a brief temporary felicity is derived at the expense of subsequent long drawn out misery and disease."[17] "Artificial tastes" and "depraved appetites" are how the Standard American Diet has come to be for Kellogg, with its reliance on salt and processed foods: "The addition of salt to the food is necessary only to please an artificial taste."[18] It is only a return to nature through the rejection of adulteration that can restore taste to its regulatory function.

In a state of unmediated existence with nature, Kellogg argues, humans will self-regulate. But it is an unfortunate effect of civilization that human tastes have become increasingly distant from the animal instincts that guided humanity through its earliest eras. Kellogg explicitly associates humans with their nonhuman animal cousins, who, for him, exist in a closer relationship with nature and its cues:

> It is unbelievable that the human race has from the beginning been inferior to animals in the ability to select the foods necessary to meet nutritive requirements; but somewhere on the long road from our prehistoric origin down to our present degenerated state, this food-regulating instinct has been to such a degree obliterated or blunted that . . . it was supposed to be lost. Indeed, it cannot be denied that man's best performance in this line is highly inferior to what is seen in lower animals, for the wolf, the monkey, and wild animals generally, and to a very large extent domestic animals, determine the wholesomeness of food by the senses of smell and taste; but in man this power is so nearly lost that be derives comparatively little assistance from his senses in the selection of food with reference to its healthful properties. It is quite possible, however, that future investigations may show that the olfactory and the gustatory nerves which are closely associated in the sensations we call taste, may be the seat of wonderful reflexes through which the body may govern the intake of new material so as best to meet its essential needs.[19]

The use of "govern" here ties taste to the regulatory powers of the body, an intrinsic capacity of animal life that civilization has come to interfere with. Humans, Kellogg suggests, would do well to attend to their nonhuman cousins in ascertaining what their actual needs are and how they might be met. The senses play a critical role in maintaining health as a homeostatic state; smell and taste provide an individual's body with the information it needs in order to meet its "healthful" acquisition of nutrients, and when the senses become perverted due to a desire for the "pleasures of the table," the senses lead the body astray through perverted tastes. Those pleasures, while they may be temporarily seductive, lead to a growing gap between our animal ways of knowing the world and meeting our body's needs and what we seek out to meet our desires. It is here that he focuses attention on "perversion" as a way to understand how our base natures have become so distant from what they should be.

In a section of *The Stomach* entitled "Perverted Appetites," Kellogg recognizes that what might appear to be a divergence from the body's needs is based, initially, in a natural logic of meeting the body's physiological requirements. Thus, a practice that begins because it meets an instinctual, animal need—as in the sufficient consumption of a particular vitamin or mineral—can result in a pathological eating behavior that is structured as a habit. In the example that Kellogg provides to explore this, he explicitly compares tribal peoples of the Americas with "young women, chiefly schoolgirls." Such a comparison implicitly trades in racism and sexism, producing "young women" as driven by the same natural instincts as the Indigenous "tribes" of the Americas, which he ascribes to a less civilized status:

> Strangely perverted tastes, as shown in a fondness for earthy and other inorganic or innutritions substances, while sometimes the result of dyspepsia, are often the cause of stomach disorders. They are either the result of nervous or mental disease, or are adopted as a habit through example. In South America there are whole tribes of human beings who habitually eat considerable quantities of a peculiar kind of clay. Several North American tribes have the same habit, being known as clay-eaters. A similar propensity sometimes appears among more civilized human beings, being almost exclusively confined, however, to young women, chiefly schoolgirls, who acquire the habit of chewing up slate pencils, and gradually become so fond of such earthy substances that they have in some instances been known to eat very considerable quantities of chalk, clay, and similar substances. While indicating a depraved state of the system, and often of the mind also, this practice has a very pernicious effect upon the stomach, which is not intended, as is that of the fowl, to receive inorganic matter of that sort.[20]

The use of "depraved state of the system, and often of the mind also" indexes the depth of the perversion, which may begin with a physiological need but becomes concretized as a "habit" with its own compulsions. The result, Kellogg suggests, is both a form of mental illness, as captured in the compulsive consumption of something that is not food, and a physical illness, as the stomach "is not intended" to take on raw minerals in the same way that some avian species have evolved. Civilization is useful in providing necessary elements of the diet through agriculture, but a perverse civilization is one that has diverged from a basic physiological need toward the provision and consumption of too much of a necessary thing, or something unnecessary altogether. As a set of socialized eating habits, civilization compels consumption and creates tastes for the "pleasures of the table" that may be at odds with the stomach and its functioning, resulting in ill health. For Kellogg, overcoming these habits and the civilized tastes that make us ill requires adopting a diet that is based in foods that meet our physiological needs and a schedule that regulates our bodies in ways that produce a natural rhythm.

Fundamentally, Kellogg argues that human eating practices should be based in a vegetarian diet, tied to the natural rhythms of the land and its productive powers. What Kellogg refers to as "animal foods," meaning meat and dairy products, are an outgrowth of early civilizations that have only intensified over time, serving as one of the vectors through which humans have become divorced from their physiological needs. A taste for animal products leads to the consumption of materials that rot in the gut, creating the condition of autointoxication; a vegetable-based diet moves through the body more quickly, avoiding the process of rot. In a precursor to contemporary interests in "raw food" diets, Kellogg writes that: "Vegetable foods taken in a raw or uncooked state are digested before it is possible for them to undergo destructive changes, and thus their use discourages the growth of bacteria in the intestine, especially those of the putrefactive sort."[21] It is in these ways that nonhuman animals and "primitive savages" are more robust than "civilized man," as he writes: "The beasts of the forest, and to a large extent also the primitive savage, take their food directly from the hands of nature, unsophisticated and uninjured, and as result enjoy an immunity from disease and acquire a vigor and toughness of constitution which are unknown to civilized man."[22] The conflation of "beasts of the forest" and "primitive savage" imply race as a means to denigrate Kellogg's contemporary readers who understand their eating to have become perverted in some way. They may not be eating clay, but the implication is that what may have begun as a means to meet a physiological need has become a habit resulting in poor health. Cultivating a sense of disgust provides a means to reject the "pleasures of the table," which Kellogg captures in a brief diatribe against the use of adulterating condiments: "None of the several food elements [condiments] which we have been considering are, in any proper sense, to be regarded as food. An animal fed exclusively on any one of them soon acquires such a disgust for its food that it will refuse to taste it, even though starving, and sooner or later dies."[23] As a capacity, Kellogg casts "disgust" as a feature of animal life; humans are likely to disguise their capacity for disgust through the selective eating of things without nutritional value. When this dietary choice is compounded with the use of condiments (Kellogg portrays the excessive use of salt as an example), people can find themselves consuming a diet made up of food that is not "true food." A finer attunement to one's physiological capacity of disgust provides the basis for resisting the forces that lead to individual and race degeneracy.

## Race Degeneracy and the Problems of Civilization

Kellogg believes that taste and pleasure are the vehicles through which race degeneracy occurs. This is a passive form of eugenics, but one that is shaped by the tastes that have been forwarded through the tacit acceptance of foodways that are part of cultural traditions.[24] Through one's inattention to what is being eaten, and often being duped by a cultivated sense of taste that chafes against nutritional needs, an individual falls into disease, leading potentially to kin and community falling prey to disease as well. But the individual is the vector through which this corruption occurs, and it is the choices that they make that lead first to individual disease, and eventually "race degeneracy." As a form of eugenics, race degeneracy is one that places responsibility on the individual and their care of the self; it draws its moral strength from the scaling between the individual and their obligation to their "race." Throughout his work, Kellogg is careful in his use of racial markers, rarely using then-contemporary terms like "Negro" and "Indian," and instead relying on terms like "savage" and "primitive." It is a canny form of racism that works through implication.

In its way, it operates through instilling a need to cultivate oneself away from an inner savage or primitive, balanced against the impulses of civilization that lead to corruption. Whiteness exists in that space of self-regulation. "Pleasure" is what must be regulated against, as it is the means through which civilization's excesses enter the body.

> Eating must not be regarded as a pastime, as a means of pleasurable diversion or entertainment. For many generations the palate has been made a source of pleasure, and to the great detriment of the race. A large share of the physical degeneracy that is increasing on every hand may be traced directly to improper eating, to the eating of things never designed to be eaten, and which no one would ever think of eating, except for that fact that they momentarily give an agreeable sensation to the tongue and palate.[25]

The challenge, as Kellogg portrays it, is overcoming the "momentary" individual pleasures one experiences in order to act against the forces of racial corruption. Because taste has been corrupted, substituting innutritious foods for ones that meet our physiological needs, our pleasures cannot be trusted. These fleeting moments of pleasure are captured in Kellogg's analogy of the human body as a harp to be played, its strings vibrating with pleasure only as long as they are plucked: "While man regards his body as a harp of pleasure to be played upon so long as its strings can be made to vibrate, so long will he continue to travel down the hill of physical decadence and degeneration in spite of quarantine laws and the most minute sanitary regulations."[26] Modest injunctions on behavior, like "minute sanitary regulations," serve as ways to shape one's pleasure-seeking but require an individual to self-regulate. The law, religion, or whatever form the injunction takes—"repression," in Bourke's terms—must be inhabited by the individual, cultivating a sensibility of pleasure-avoidance.

One's "savage" insides can be known through one's bodily rhythms. If constipation is a malady associated with the rhythms and diets of modern civilization and regular, timely bowel movements are associated with an intimacy with nature that is demonstrated by uncivilized people, then constipation in a civilized person is a clear marker that a person has become too distant from one's inner nature. Balancing oneself between the unmediated "savage" and the corrupt modern eater becomes possible through attention to one's bodily rhythms. Kellogg portrays the problem and possibility in this way:

> Savages rarely suffer from constipation, which is also true of the more primitive of so-called civilized nations. Chronic intestinal inactivity is much less frequent among country people than among those living in the city. It is manifestly a morbid condition peculiar to a state of high civilization; and modern medical researches tend to show that this condition and its results may justly be looked upon as among the fundamental causes of the race degeneracy which is becoming every year more apparent in all highly civilized communities.[27]

Constipation provides both an individual diagnostic and a societal one, providing a means for Kellogg to scale from the individual to the "race." The blight of constipation shows both how an individual's wellness has diverged from the possibilities of being in tune with nature and how civilization has diverged from nature and its implicit regulation of human bodies through diet and activity tied to the land and its productivity. Such societal collapse can be recognized in the rise of chronic illnesses, which are a product of the autointoxication that results from constipation; the widespread phenomena of constipation leads, in time, to diminished immune functioning and the eventual end of a race: "Increase of chronic disease is a certain indication of race degeneration, since it indicates diminished power of resistance to the death dealing conditions with which man's environment in civilized life bring him in daily contact."[28]

Yet it is not solely one's diet that leads to constipation, autointoxication, and chronic illness. The very organizing structures of everyday life compel ill health, which is evident in how our individual bodies respond to their natural cues. In this respect, bowel movements provide Kellogg with a further way to promote attention to self-regulation against an imagined "savage":

> With the savage, regularity of bowel movement is not a matter of so great importance, for the reason that he is rarely so situated that he cannot respond quickly to the "call" for evacuation. But civilized human beings by their systematic and, in general, their closely occupied life, must often find themselves in circumstances which compel

a considerable delay in answering the "call" without being seriously incommoded.[29]

"Regularity" here is a function of proximity to nature, where "delay" results from a form of social organization ("business" and capitalism) wherein the "call for evacuation" must be ignored, leading to knock-on effects on one's health. Humans can depend on a regularity supplied by nature and embodied in their everyday practice, but their competing dependence on civilization and its demands interrupts this regularity, demanding a form of self-regulation that embraces a model of natural rhythm provided by the precivilized savage.

If Kellogg's racism were strictly related to his imagination of a noble savage and primordial humanity, it might be relatively benign. Where his racism bites hardest is in his association of particular people with animals, a form of comparison that attributes nonhuman capacities to groups of people as a means to tie them more closely with nonhuman animals. This occurs both in the association of physiological qualities with specific people and in the attribution of uncivilized or precivilized practices to groups. He attributes a power of digestion to the "negro of the Nile and the Bushman" that is possible for any human to have, but the "civilized" whites of Europe and North America have lost. He here compares people of Africa to herbivorous animals:

> It is well known that the digestive organ of herbivorous animals are [*sic*] able to digest cellulose, a function which seems to have been lost by civilized human beings, for it has been shown ... that the capacious cecum of the negro of the Nile and the Bushman secretes a ferment which dissolves the cellulose covering of vegetable cells. It is claimed, also, that the vermiform appendix of the negro produces a ferment which digests cellulose.[30]

It is not that Kellogg argues for an innate physiological difference between one group of people and another that constitutes his racism. Rather, the combined association of peoples of diverse parts of Africa with nonhuman animals and their association with uncorrupted nature serve as a means to situate Blackness as outside of whiteness. For Kellogg, whiteness can contain Blackness within it, and likewise Blackness can be cultivated to become more white, but they are fundamentally different due to their situation as civilized and natural, respectively. In a more mundane fashion, Kellogg argues that something as everyday as drinking with a meal is something that "primitive" people do not do, marking their practical difference from civilized people—and their attunement to a natural form of digestive regulation. "Neither tea and coffee nor any other harmful or intoxicating drink was indulged by the aborigines of this country [the United States], although they made many agreeable beverages from the pulp of fruits of various sorts. These primitive people, like the wild animals which shared the forests with them, refrained from drinking at meals, as do all primitive people."[31] There is barely space between "primitive people" and "wild animals" in this analogy, associating the precivilized with the untamed; that Kellogg directly associates native North Americans with wild animals in this way is explicitly racist. His racism is associated with their practices, themselves a benign marker of difference between the savage and civilized. This facilitates his implicit belief that, through a change of practices, a person might become more white; they might become more civilized. In so doing, a person runs the risk of falling into the pleasure-seeking regulation of civilization and its adulterated and adulterating tastes and outside nature's rhythms and regulation.

It is this adoption of practice as the basis for racialization that moves from individual poor health to race degeneracy and the fall of nations, balancing whiteness individually and socially on the precipice of pleasure and necessity. Avoiding the pitfalls of pleasure, Kellogg suggests, is necessarily an individual practice, and one that relies on a cultivation of habit. "Purity of the mind is a condition quite incompatible with gluttonous habits of eating. The pages of history are crowded with facts which clearly show that the successive degeneracy of each of the nations which ruled the world, began with luxuriousness in diet."[32] That "purity" plays a role here indexes Kellogg's conception of how taste must operate for individuals in order to uphold the needs of one's race: one's habit must not only ensure individual health, but also ensures a purity of being that is reflected in society as a whole. Scaling up to all of American society and the "race decay" that it faces suggests to Kellogg that "all civilized races" are degenerating, an implicit construction of a failing whiteness that has given itself over to the "pleasures of the table." He writes: "That the human race is degenerating, at least that there is a decided trend toward race deterioration going on among all civilized races, is no longer disputed. . . . The civilized portion of the human race is showing many most decided evidences of race decay."[33] The responsibility to act against the slow tides of race degeneracy falls to the individual and the remaking of regular habits.

The remedies for this race degeneration are based in a return to nature, both in relation to one's eating habits and in a return to prelapserian nature and its rhythms more generally. On one level, this motivates a return to a vegetarian diet that ensures a regular set of bowel movements over a day; on another level, it means a societal embrace of a return to a less urban, less "civilized" way of life, one that accepts the possibility of the savage within as the basis for a form of wellness that exceeds the "pleasures of the table" and their temporary indulgences.

> The remedy proposed is to bring every child into actual contact with the real and natural life of the land, from which our modern civilization has so far divorced us, and by this means to antagonize to as great an extent as possible both the mental and the physical perversions which are the natural results of city life and which are doubtless the chief factors in modern race deterioration.[34]

Kellogg's assumption is that only a genuine reconnection with nature can overcome the forces of civilization that have divorced individuals from their physiological needs and restore the natural forms of regulation that ensure needs are being met in healthy and sustainable ways. His call for a return to nature is not a unique one, but rather a widely shared view of the corrupting forces of modern life in the United States in an era of rapid urbanization and its effects on individual health, including epidemic disease, pollution, and sedentariness.[35] His call for a return to nature echoes today and is reflected, in quite different ways, in ideas about diets and microbial medicine. And as Kellogg knew, the microbial offered the promise of health, but his view of how it could be acted on trafficked in his conceptions of purity and diet that shaped the rest of his thought.

## Putrefaction unto Death

For Kellogg, the human body is a vessel, shaped by the contents that one puts into it. But it is not an entirely neutral vessel, and it is likely to be influenced not only by the contents, but by how the contents are processed and their byproducts. This is captured, above, in his view that vegetables move through the body without fermentation, yet meat decomposes in the digestive tract and produces "toxins" that "intoxicate" the body. Constipation too produces this process of autointoxication, leading to disease—and, across society, to racial degeneration. As a vessel, the human body is a precarious one, subject to disease through consumption and subject to degeneration through its practices, leading to a slide from the civilized to the savage, a loss of a cultivated whiteness that is balanced between nature and civilization. While his racial logics of corruption and his basic nutritive understanding of foodstuff are both misguided, he captures an emerging conception of the microbial and its potentials in his interests in the unseen and its effects on human health. Kellogg captures the microbial threats to the body in a discussion of fermentation and putrefaction:

> We may say that fermentation germs feed upon vegetable and putrefaction germs upon animal substances. . . . Fermentation germs produce for the most part acids, especially lactic and acetic acids, which, in the small quantities in which they are produced in the body, are practically harmless. Putrefaction germs, on the other hand, produce by the decomposition of proteins, especially when acting upon animal proteins, highly poisonous toxins, many of which closely resemble the venom of snakes and which are capable of producing in the most minute quantities the most alarming and distressing symptoms.[36]

Kellogg's awareness of the "minute quantities" of substances influencing health structures his imagination about how porous the body is, not only in the foods one eats but in one's exposures more generally. This is the basis for his call for a return to a finer relationship with nature, but also his emergent sense of public health and the influences one body has on others. In the following, he captures his fears of putrefying flesh with a sense of interpersonal disgust, a disgust that is not just about other people's bodies, but what their bodies bring to public spaces and their impingement on the health of others:

> The bowel discharges of a meat-eater, exposed in a closed room, would in an hour or two render the place intolerable, even to a very robust person. . . . If the mere breathing of the greatly diluted volatile poisons

arising from such putrescent matter will produce highly unpleasant effects, how much more grave must be the effects when through the retention within the body of these foul substances all of their poisonous contents are absorbed and sucked up into the blood and circulated throughout the body![37]

Such a conception of bodies and their processes skirts the microbial; it accepts that the odors that our bodies emit are not just unpleasant smells, but part of a corrupting process of one's digesting body, and a means to affect other bodies. The microbial is buried there, an understanding of the invisible influences on human health that exceed food itself. As close as he comes to a conception of microbial medicine, Kellogg largely backs away from it, accepting in the processes of fermentation and putrefaction dangers to the individual and society. He writes in his most definitive stance against the microbial that: "It is now clearly established that we do not live by the aid of the germs that throng our intestines and swarm upon the surface of the body, but rather that we live in spite of these microbic enemies."[38]

Yet, microbial medicine was possible. Elsewhere in Kellogg's corpus he recognizes that microbes can be beneficial and that they might even be used as a medical therapeutic. In the following, he understands the role of the intestinal flora in determining health and also provides an early conception of a restricted diet to enhance the flora through selective consumption. It is a diet that will return in the form of the GAPS diet ("gut and psychological syndrome"), at which point (chapter 6) the connection between the colony within and more general states of health will be more fully articulated. Here, though, Kellogg lays the groundwork for exclusion diets and their role in shaping the intestinal flora, including the use of fermented milk in the form of buttermilk.

> It is possible to change the intestinal flora, and that this change is one of the most practical and important means of combating the great majority of the chronic diseases with which the physician has to deal. A method which has been thoroughly tested is the following: . . . The adoption of a strict antitoxic diet. This requires, for most rapid results, the exclusion of all animal protein; that is, meat, including fish, fowl and game, as well as beef, mutton and pork, together with eggs and

milk and all preparations and dishes containing these animal proteins must be strictly avoided. In extreme cases of autointoxication, the strict exclusion of all animal protein is absolutely necessary. In milder cases milk, especially in the form of buttermilk, may be used.[39]

The most potentially revolutionary of Kellogg's insights comes elsewhere though, in his discussion of the use of a "special culture" as the basis of enema to change the intestinal flora. While not using human excrement as medicine, his use of the microbes that ferment milk into yogurt, *Bacillus bulgaricus,* is microbial medicine and verges on the technology that fecal microbial transplantation offers. He writes, suggestively, that:

> Of great value in special cases, particularly in cases of spastic constipation due to colitis, is a measure by means of which change of the flora may be greatly expedited by introducing the special culture [*Bacillus bulgaricus*], . . . along with milk sugar or malt sugar, into the colon. . . . The culture is usually administered at night and is if possible retained over night so as to give opportunity for the growth and development of the acid-forming organisms in the colon.[40]

Kellogg was on the cusp of the microbial in medicine, but potentially was too influenced by his conceptions of degeneration, both in the form of food putrefying in the body and in racial degeneration, which motivated his sense of disgust. As a physician, he would largely become eclipsed by industrial biomedicine, which favored the increasing use of pharmaceuticals to affect the illnesses that Kellogg thought of as being able to be addressed through exercise, diet, and self-regulation. Pharmaceuticals would produce a regulation of their own, offloading the need to self-regulate into "compliance"; but Kellogg offered another possibility in shaping human health through a focus on diet. It is this legacy of purifying one's body through one's diet that lays the basis for the natural-foods movement in the twentieth century, which similarly saw a return to nature as beneficial for the individual and society. But a return to nature in this way also came to include, specifically, a return to the microbial in ways that Kellogg could only indirectly accept.

Instead of accepting that substances might be a primary vehicle for changing the health of individuals, Kellogg relied on ideas about habit and its spatiotemporally structuring effects as a means for intervention into individual well-being. Habit, for Kellogg and many of his peers, served as a means to create the conditions whereby one's health could be maintained.[41] As a form of self-regulation, habits serve as everyday means to manage the body, from daily hygiene practices to the timing and content of meals, to exercise and practices of rest and sleep.[42] Ideally, when practiced in line with the prescriptions that proponents provide, habits can serve as prophylactic against disease. This is the basis for American health-related self-help practices, which often come paired with necessary changes in what people consume and how they consume it. The problem with habits is that they can be subject to outside forces, which makes them fundamentally precarious. As American ideas about dieting and parenting developed in the twentieth century (which comprises my focus for chapters 3 and 4), habit became a central feature in how Americans imagine practices influencing the health outcomes for adults and children. In this way, habits are the bodily substantiation of self-regulation, and a well-regulated person will abide by habits that shape an individual in distinct ways that are aligned with the spatiotemporal demands of one's social world. But, when habits are inexact in their effects or misaligned with a person's needs, reforming one's habits provides a mechanism to realign with the normative demands of the biology of everyday life.

# 3 Cultivating the Taste for Whiteness
## YOGURT, ADULTERATION, AND EUGENIC THINKING

IF JOHN HARVEY KELLOGG represented dominant American attitudes about the microbial in the early twentieth century as a negative byproduct of an unhealthy diet, Adelle Davis slowly worked to expand the conceptions of the health benefits of microbial agents. This occurred throughout Davis's corpus of cookbooks and self-help books, which spanned the 1920s through 1970s, with reprints and updated versions of her books appearing through the present. She is one of the most widely circulated lay nutritionists of the twentieth century, with covers of her books from the 1970s proclaiming that she has sold over ten million books, and an enduring Adelle Davis Foundation that continues to promote her work. Davis may be one of the most quietly influential nutritionists of the twentieth century, her ideas having shaped the natural-foods movement of the 1960s, reflected in cookbooks produced by the Rodale Institute,[1] the Moosewood collective, and more recent diet authors, all of whom emphasize the importance of microbial elements in food or the inclusion of "ethnic" foods as essential to natural foodways. Many of these "ethnic" elements were fermented foods: sauerkraut, pickles, kefir, and as I discuss in detail in this chapter, yogurt. These foods have become "probiotics" and include kimchi, kombucha, and other fermented foodstuff, all of which trouble Kellogg's understanding of the dangers of fermented materials in the body. But the challenge natural-food cookbook authors faced was shaping American tastes to accept the strange flavors that fermented foods presented; ultimately, much of what natural food writers advocated for would become adulterated through food processing to make it palatable to American consumers. Yogurt is exemplary in this way, having become established in the U.S. food market through a combination of persistence and adaptation to American desires.

In this chapter, I first focus on Davis and her contributions to American nutritional thought and practice, situating her as a token of a broader movement that focused on the acceptance of natural foods and their place in the American diet against the elements of the Standard American Diet, which she treats as a foil. In this respect, Davis carried the torch for Kellogg, continuing to argue for the return to nature that Kellogg called for; what differed was that Davis's conception of what "natural" foods included was significantly different from Kellogg's and incorporated many of the foodways that were once thought of as "ethnic." Davis's success is based in her ability to appeal to familiarity, building off foods that people know and are comfortable with in ways that extend the boundaries of individual diets. Throughout her corpus, she is invested in convincing her readers to do things "right," working against traditional practices that they have habitually accepted in order to create more nutritious meals. In this way, she extends Kellogg's interests in habit to lay the foundation for individuals to incorporate new foods and practices into their diets so as to achieve better health. Davis's thought, like Kellogg's, is influenced by euthenics, the eugenic attempt to modify living conditions—including foodways—in order to achieve better individual outcomes, scalable to the family, community, and nation. Like with Kellogg, individual health is fundamentally an individual concern for her, but Davis accepts that some inclusion of the microbial can alter one's well-being, marking her difference from Kellogg.

Writing about Davis and the emergence of the natural-foods movement in the United States is an intimate history for me. Raised by a natural-food-loving mother, for whom Rodale cookbooks were steady resources in the kitchen, I was exposed to organic "health" foods from a very early age, as they formed the foundation of our household diet. This led, throughout my youth, to curiosity about the foods that other people were eating: mass-produced, mainstream foods were alien, which often propelled me through binges of Doritos at sleepovers. As a young adult, when it came time to determine my diet for myself, I struggled with the tensions between the costs associated with the diet I was raised on and the appetites it created; it led me to train myself to cook, which itself was built on a foundation laid by my mother and her inclusion of me and my brother in preparing family meals. Cuisine by cuisine, I taught myself basic techniques and use of ingredients, and when it came time to cook for my family, I found myself reproducing in spirit if not in substance the meals my mother prepared for us as children. Because of this, the New American Diet is one that is proximate to me, with embedded assumptions about the Standard American Diet; the history of American natural-foods movements is proximate too, as it dovetails with my family history. At times, it is an uncomfortable history, as the foundations of the natural-food movement run through troubling racist and eugenicist attitudes toward people and their foods, as in the case of yogurt.

In the early and mid-twentieth century, yogurt, for Davis and mainstream white Americans, existed on the edges of the Standard American Diet. Yogurt is similar to already-accepted foods as a milk product, yet it is different enough that Davis felt it needed to be advocated for in order to be accepted as part of everyday eating. Yogurt's challenge is that it carries "ethnic" baggage, a result of the commonly told folk tales about its origins and existence in the United States, the result of immigration from southeastern Europe and the Middle East. Yogurt was "not quite white" in the early twentieth century, and it was ultimately through its adulteration with sugar and fruits that it became mainstream, rather than an ethnic food or part of a fad diet through which advertisers sought to appeal to women. In telling the history of the Colombosian family in this chapter and their marketing of Colombo yogurt in the early–mid twentieth century, a critical element of the story is how yogurt became "white" as white ethnics became white, an effect of changing political contexts, suburbanization, and labor movements in the United States. To be clear, yogurt did not become "white" because ethnic whites did; instead, through a parallel process of commodification and adulteration, yogurt became a commodity in much the same way that ethnic whites became mainstreamed into American society as laborers, politicians, and full members of society—they both became naturalized by becoming objects of American capital.[2]

Yogurt provides an example for how many Americans come to cultivate a taste for difference. To be sure, it is a difference that is curated for them, adulterated with sugar and fruit, marketed as low fat and slimming;

yogurt was made to fit into a set of American desires about bodies and their tastes, so as not to be too different. As its popularity grew, yogurt could become more diverse and appeal to more consumers. One way this occurred was in the marketing of yogurt as a "probiotic," a food technology to heal the body from within. The appeal to yogurt's healing properties was a recurrent one, extending, with some frequency, throughout the twentieth century; its foreignness provided the possibility of something unexpected (good health), but it needed to be shaped in order to appeal to American tastes. In the following, yogurt provides a token of changing American tastes, how they become enrolled in ideas about nature and health, and how, together, they conjure a framework for conceptualizing microbial medicine and its acceptance in American society. Central to all of this is a recentering of disgust, which, Kellogg and John Bourke portray as a reaction to the other; but if it is instead situated in the self, this provides a therapeutic process to overcome in self-care. Not to make too much of this transition, but one might accept it as reflective of broader attitudes to race and racism in the United States, moving toward a conception of tolerance for the benefit of society in the context of growing multiculturalism and changing contours of whiteness in the post–World War II American society.[3]

"Cultivation," as Kellogg and Davis portray it, is based in nature; it assumes that there is a natural capacity for something and that, through careful action, that capacity can be increased. It provides a foil for "acquisition," which assumes that there is a void and that something can be put into its place. Cultivating taste, for Davis, is an attempt to realign the individual with nature. If our tastes are neutral and something we acquire over time, they are also plastic and able to be shaped by environmental and social influences. The problem that Davis diagnoses, much like Kellogg, is that Americans have lost their taste for natural foods and have instead become dependent on processed foods, which are nutritionally unfulfilling. And so, cultivating taste for the natural means embracing foods that taste different from what many Americans have come to desire and eating foods that meet the physiological needs of their bodies. Like Kellogg's before it, Davis's work has an undercurrent of racism in it, an euthenics-based conception that changing one's environment can lead to the enhancement of individual lives and whole societies, and that degeneracy can occur through individual poor diets and the poor diets of whole communities. She is careful throughout her work to avoid language about race, but her references to "welfare" and urban populations who are sliding into violence and disease make her politics plain. The implication is that, to end cycles of poverty, violence, and disease, it is insufficient to just eat "right"; one must also eat "white," embodied in the natural-foods movement and its emerging embrace of the microbial.

"Adulteration" is a key metaphor, alongside cultivation, and extends Kellogg's attitudes toward food additives to the growing American food market in the middle twentieth century. As Bob Colombosian will suggest in my history of the introduction of yogurt into American markets, adulteration is taken as changing the fundamental nature of a substance. This may be, as in the case of yogurt, to "enhance" it, or it may be to make it palatable for a new audience of consumers. But adulteration also lurks in Davis's conception of cultivation. For Davis, our tastes have been adulterated in ways that have removed us from our natural propensities to know our bodies and their needs through taste and appetite: Americans have become adulterated through the Standard American Diet and need to cultivate a countersensibility to realign themselves with nature. In this way, adulteration is the inverse of cultivation: rather than producing "civilized" bodies and tastes, it produces the artificial as a problem to be overcome. Habits step in here and provide the means to counteract adulteration through the careful development of practices of self-regulation based in a sense of disgust in the artificial. But, as the history of yogurt also shows, adulteration can provide a gateway for consumers to find their way toward the unadulterated, "natural" form of a food, itself a form of deliberate cultivation that may require unsettling one's disgust.

## The Racial Logic of "Natural Foods"

Many natural-food writers in the early twentieth century, like Davis, were inspired by the work of Weston Price, a dentist who traveled the world in an attempt to catalogue the deteriorating impacts of civilization on human health. Price, much like Kellogg, saw contemporary diets and lifeways as interrupting a natural relationship between humans and their environments, reflected in the foods they ate and the diseases people in

North America and Europe were exhibiting. And, as it did for Kellogg, this motivated a concern with eugenics, reflected in Price's use of "race betterment." This is captured in the following, where he pits the individual decisions that lead to disease against the drive on the part of health-care providers to combat these emerging illnesses: "Modern civilization is in a dilemma. The biggest problem in the world today is not war, but means for race betterment. Epidemics, plagues and infectious diseases are largely under control. Today, the members of the healing professions are engaged in alleviating suffering from degenerative diseases by means of remedial surgery and makeshift repairs."[4] Like Kellogg and other health reformers in the early twentieth century, Price saw food as a primary influence in deteriorating human health, which could be appreciated through an examination of individual dental health, a method that Kellogg embraced as well. As Kellogg writes, betraying his racist conceptions of nature: "The teeth of Orientals, negroes, and in fact of nearly all primitive people, are generally remarkably sound, because of their simpler diet and small use of meat."[5] Kellogg elaborates, elsewhere, what the effects of tooth decay wrought by civilized diets lead to:

> The microbes harbored by decaying teeth are swept into the stomach in drinking or eating, and there set up fermentative and putrefactive processes, whereby the food elements are converted into poisonous substances. Some of these poisons are possessed of such strong odors as to taint the breath. Decaying teeth may also be the means of introducing into the body such destructive microbes as the germs of consumption, and others giving rise to serious and even fatal disease.[6]

Such a conception of dental health finds in the untouched and undecayed teeth of "primitive people" the basis for claims that a diet more attuned to nature will enhance health; whether dental health among "primitive people" was as high as Kellogg and Price portray it, the claim provided a foundation, as a foil to civilized mouths, to argue against the ills of a highly processed diet. In this way, knowing one's teeth is a means to knowing one's diet as well, including the elements that may be invisible—those "harbored" microbes putrefying the body from within.[7]

For Price, then-contemporary Indigenous groups provided a glimpse of a prelapsarian equilibrium with nature, one that was knowable through their healthiness and based in their natural diets. With esteem for a form of precivilized life that allowed individuals to "build superb bodies," Price writes of Indigenous people in North America: "Primitive Indians living in that very inclement climate were able, before the advent of the modern foods, to build superb bodies and that, in even the first generation after the arrival of modern foods, their children broke down with typical nutritional deficiency diseases."[8] Price associates the decline of health specifically with "modern foods," which, writing originally in the 1930s, would accord closely with the recent introduction of manufactured foods like canned fruits, vegetables, and meats and industrially produced breads. Such foods offered consumers convenience, but also a break from the natural rhythms of agriculture and the seasonal foods that a more nature-attuned lifeway might provide, however impossible such a life was becoming as a result of suburbanization and industrialization, as well as the effects of the Depression and World War II. Echoing Kellogg, Price writes: "We do not realize how much modern human beings are handicapped and injured since they learned how to modify Nature's foods. The wild animal uses Nature's foods as Nature makes them. This was true of the earlier races of mankind. In proportion as man has learned to modify Nature's foods, he has degenerated."[9] As it did for Kellogg, "race degeneration" motivated Price too, a fall from the grace of nature and the food it provided. Although Price's followers in the natural-food movement distanced themselves, implicitly, from his concerns with "race degeneration" and the fantasy of "primitive people" attuned to the natural world, they often accepted, explicitly, that more "natural" foods that were less processed were integral to human health, and that a return to a more attuned relationship with nature through consumption was a vital means to restore individual health, if not the health of the nation.[10]

In this respect, Davis's recommendations for health are relatively straightforward. She prizes unadulterated foods, and accepts that a diet high in fruits, vegetables, dairy, and grains, largely in the form of bread, is key to a healthy body.[11] Throughout her work, she is concerned with changing American tastes, toiling against ingrained forms of disgust with food that might seem strange to many American eaters. This is vital because, in addition to ingredients and foods that Americans might find ordinary and part of an everyday diet, Davis is interested in introducing eaters to the possibilities of more natural foods, especially including brewer's yeast and yogurt, due to their promotion of the creation of vitamin B12, which she accepts as essential to digestion. Later in her career, Davis became associated with "supervitaminization," the macrodosing of industrially produced vitamin supplements. This was an extension of a set of beliefs she held throughout her writing career about natural processes that found their roots in the increased scientific knowledge about vitamins as components of foods, their physiological extraction and production, and their effects on human health.[12] Her promotion of vitamins tracks the rise of the natural-food movement into the mainstream in the 1960s and demonstrates how an interest in scientific knowledge about foods and their impacts on the human body provided the foundation for a new form of appeal to nature: earlier ideologies about what constituted natural foods because of their lack of processing fell alongside the construction of foods as being natural because of their effects on the human body. Natural foods had nature-enhancing effects on bodies.

For Davis, the promotion of an emergent American sense of taste based in health-promoting foods was beset by American consumers' interests in foods that appealed to their extant sense of taste, much like Kellogg's "pleasures of the table." As an example of this, her discussion of the merits of cow milk in *Let's Cook It Right,* which she describes as "beautifully white,"[13] is illustrative. Davis is committed to milk as a natural, health-promoting substance and attempts to situate it as better than water because of its nutrient value, but has to additionally work against the industrial adulteration of milk to make it more than a natural substance.[14] She argues: "Milk is such a valuable food that a quart daily should be drunk by each person, regardless of age. . . . One should learn to enjoy the taste of milk and drink it with meals and between meals, as a substitute for water."[15] She goes on to argue against chocolate milk, which is associated with poor health and a symbolic foil to the "beautiful" whiteness of unadulterated milk. "A form of milk which cannot be recommended is chocolate milk. . . . Experiments have shown that animals fed chocolate milk absorbed less calcium and phosphorus than did animals given plain milk; their growth was retarded, and their bones were much smaller and more fragile."[16] Davis's rationale for her disregard of chocolate milk is based in a nutrient-level euthenics thinking, but it traffics in a politics of purity that relies on the symbolic association of whiteness with purity and darkness (here, chocolate) with danger. And that danger is not restricted to an individual's health; such safety is critical to maintain for the whole of society.

In *Let's Eat Right to Keep Fit,* Davis scales between individual choices about food, their effects on a person's well-being, and what she accepts as a threat to American society. As a form of hyperbole, her rhetorical appeal for "right" eating rails against a diverse set of dangers in midcentury American everyday life, from processed foods to open warfare.

> When the blood sugar is extremely low, the resulting irritability, nervous tension, and mental depression are such that a person can easily go berserk. If hatred, bitterness, and resentments are harbored, and perhaps a temporary psychological upset causes a person to go on a candy binge or makes it impossible for him to eat or digest food, the stage is set; violence or quarreling can occur for which there may be no forgiving. Add a few guns, gas jets, or razor blades, and you have the stuff murders and suicides are made of. The American diet has become dangerous in more ways than one.[17]

The stakes for an individual's diet are high for Davis: the potential for a missed meal or an innutritious one resulting in "extremely low" blood sugar—a physiological effect of an individual choice—scales up to shape affect, leading to the possibility that a person could "easily go berserk." Over time, the potential is that these decisions and affects are compounded, leading to ongoing health complaints, interfering with the digestion of food itself. That interruption of a basic physiological process tips into the potential for violence that is directed at the self, in suicide as an intensification of the euthenics of poor eating, and also violence directed at others, from interpersonal acts of murder to societal acts of war, captured in her use of "guns" and "gas jets."

In a 1976 edition of the same text, Davis updates these concerns to reflect growing antipathy toward urban poverty, offering an early form of blaming the victims of American divestments in urban communities, which, as a result of white flight, were becoming increasingly Black.[18] In a bid to support sentiments toward the evangelical promotion of natural foods against the use of welfare systems, she writes:

If the "solution" to the malnutrition among low-income families takes the form of welfare handouts, the American taxpayer can expect to pay doubly: first for the processed, health-destroying foods; second, for the medical care necessitated by the resulting ill-health. . . . It seems to me it is time to face the fact that producing disease in human beings is the cruelest of all possible cruelties. The amount of suffering in our nation now is astronomical. Hospitals, mental institutions, jails, drug addiction centers, all are overflowing.[19]

The racism in Davis's conception of American euthenics is implicit, as she never names racial categories of people, but it is trenchant. Her use of "low-income families" as a foil to the "American taxpayer" is a dog whistle to white Americans who fear their wages will be taxed to defray the effects of poor people's choices. If this racist appeal to taxpaying is insufficient, the moral argument she makes to end "suffering" offers a justification for the widespread push toward natural foods that seeks to act against the foodways of the urban poor. Whether Davis was aware of the growing disparities in access to food is unclear and beside the point: she is willing to blame individual actors for the choices they make, unwilling to accept the need for broad social support to change the situations individuals find themselves in, and ready to empower her readers with a sense of moral righteousness about the choices they make in their own diets and in their adherence to natural foods as an ideological commitment. This moral basis for taste provides a foundation for Davis to work on overcoming disgust as a personal experience: working through disgust to bring one closer to nature, and to well-being, becomes a moral project to work on, one meal at a time.

## Cultivating the Taste for the Microbial

Taste, for Davis, is to be "cultivated." Its foil is disgust, but disgust can be tamed in order to meet the dietary needs that individuals have. The implication, captured below in her use of "long-neglected old ones," is that what might have once been an acceptably tasty food has now fallen into the realm of disgust. Ultimately, she relies on a sense of the moral good of changing one's taste in order to break through disgust: disgust, she suggests, is not immutable and universal, but something that can be worked with in ways that provide for the possibility of acquiring the taste for something new, especially when it offers a healthy alternative to the foods one usually eats. She writes in *Let's Stay Healthy*:

> It is important to try and enjoy the taste of new foods (and some of the long-neglected old ones). You can undoubtably remember the numerous foods you disliked the first time you taste them but enjoy now. If any food can build health, set out to cultivate a taste for it. Expect to dislike it at first. Take only a small portion the first time you eat it but be prepared to try another small helping at the next opportunity. A little psychology, such as telling yourself how good the food is for you and how you are going to benefit from it, will help in the battle. You will be surprised at how soon you find you are actually enjoying the food and eating more and more of it.[20]

Portraying the cultivation of a taste for new foods as a "battle" that will result in "actual enjoyment" points to the ambivalence Davis understands as the basis of human taste. "Dislike" and enjoyment are the two reactions one might have to food and moving from one to the other is not based on an intrinsic physiological reaction, but one that is shaped by "psychology" in ways that make it mutable. "How good the food is for you and how you are going to benefit from it" provides the basis for shaping one's psychology and grounding moral claims about eating: food, in this way, is neither inherently objectionable nor appealing, but something for which taste must be shaped in order to find "actual enjoyment" in it. "Cultivating" taste becomes a moral injunction for individual eaters and for parents in their training of their children's palates so that they can be attuned to the foods that can "build health." "Right" eating is not just a process of maintaining one's bodily well-being, but a moral project that begins with the individual and extends to society; taste is the vehicle that this project operates through, which produces a form of embodied morality that begins in health and ends with the welfare of the social order. In between exist the shaping of one's body through taste and the need to shape the tastes of others as a moral project.

This is where Davis's eugenics really resides. In *Let's Raise Healthy Children,* she argues that disabilities in a child are largely due to a mother's dietary inadequacies and that, if a parent is mindful of the potential to cause "abnormalities" in their child, they will be attentive to what they eat and what they feed their child. Rather than blame poor genetics for hereditary disabilities, Davis argues that it is neglect on the part of parents that leads to their child's impairments, exposing a deep ableism:

> Large numbers of mentally retarded infants are being born daily in the United States to women lacking neither education nor money. Thousands more have IQ's within the normal range but are still far less intelligent than they should be; they have short attention spans, delayed language ability, poor social adjustment, and numerous problems related to inadequate brain development.[21]

Davis can make such claims about nutrition because she accepts that the nutrients that a child's body receives in utero are determinative of the child's development over the life-course. This can be adjusted through careful feeding once the child is born, but only within the bounds set by impairments created by a mother's unknowing neglect of a fetus and its nutritional needs. She later suggests that disease, generally, is a function of nutritional deficiencies. The cure, then, is necessarily predicated on a body receiving its required nutrients; without them, no additional medical care will be able to resolve the underlying nutritional lack.

> The important facts to remember are that the nutrients necessary to build health always remain the same regardless of a diagnosis or the nature of an abnormality; that all disease is stress, which immediately increases the need for every body requirement; and that the more quickly the diet is improved, the greater is the chance of recovery. To say that a disease is "incurable" does not mean that it cannot be cured but only that the cure is at present unknown. Since few ill children are ever allowed good nutrition, the value of an adequate diet in correcting illness is still a mystery.[22]

Her euthenics approach insists that parents take an active role in shaping the foods that children are exposed to, the nutrients they receive, and their combined impact on a child's development into an adult. This is difficult, she accepts, because agriculture in the United States has become indebted to industrial models that increasingly vacate foods of their nutritional properties and supplement poor growing conditions with pesticides, themselves toxins that are consumed by parents and children and that affect a child's development. She suggests that, with careful attention to what goes into a child's body and into the mother's body during gestation, children can become "superior." In the final paragraphs of *Let's Have Healthy Children,* she implores her reader:

> Despite faulty agricultural procedures and the overabundance of refined and processed foods, parents can still raise children with superb minds and beautiful bodies, though it is not easy. As these superior children go into the community and eventually into the world at large, their straight bodies, excellent bone structure, attractive appearance, athletic prowess, and quick grasp of social needs are all advertisements of your own efficiency as parents.[23]

The stakes for Davis are enormous, the weight on any given mother significant as they face the demands of the health of their child and the future of society. The challenge is that they are fighting against countervailing currents, besieged by industrial capitalism and its promotion of a Standard American Diet that is leading to "large numbers of mentally retarded infants" being born every day. Even after a child is born, a caregiver must remain vigilant, ensuring that the child receives the food necessary to convey vital nutrients; how this is done is through attention to individual health and the ways it can be known through physiological processes.

Individual health becomes a diagnostic to know whether one's diet is complete in fulfilling the physiological needs of the body; the process of digestion serves as a focal point in understanding whether one's body is getting what it needs, and also whether it is acting in a healthy way. This also means that restoring one's health through eating is possible and potentially desirable, serving as a means to act on the body in a pseudo-medical fashion, much like Kellogg. This is possible for Davis through a growing conception of the chemical properties of foods and their nutrient and microbial values.

> There are two approaches to improving the diet when nutrition has been neglected. The cautious approach is to increase the amounts of supplements and such foods as yeast, yogurt, or tiger's milk gradually; thereby you can prevent digestive upsets and give yourself a chance

to cultivate a taste for these foods. . . . The other approach, which can end in disaster or spectacular improvement, is to take enough supplements to saturate the tissues and large amounts of foods supplying proteins, B vitamins and other nutrients for a few days, then decrease the amount drastically when body needs have been met.[24]

"Taste" is central for Davis and serves as a means to "cultivate" an everyday practice of promoting one's well-being through the consumption of healthy foods; the alternative is the use of supplements as an emergency therapeutic. Cultivating taste is a proactive moral injunction, serving to avoid disease and also the "disaster" of requiring an infusion of supplements to counteract years of poor eating. "Right" eating for Davis—and for many food writers who followed in her wake in the natural-foods movements of the 1960s through the present—serves as a prophylactic: it ensures that one is doing as much as one can to maintain one's health. When "right" eating fails through neglect, there is always the possibility of adopting "right" eating as a means to restore health, but doing so potentially chafes against embodied taste preferences. Developing a taste for health-critical foods, like yogurt, serves as a moral project that anyone can pursue, a technology of self-making that depends on consumption with an awareness of the discreet functions of food in making a healthy body.

Yogurt, for Davis, is a novel food technology in that it can repair the body from within, based on her growing understanding of the microbial nature of fermented foods and their positive effects on individual health. In an injunction to cultivate a taste for yogurt, she writes: "If yogurt is new to you, do not expect to enjoy it immediately. Cultivate a taste for it gradually, then serve it frequently. . . . When health is below par, it is often advisable to use as much as a quart of yogurt daily, substituting it entirely for fresh milk."[25] Davis anticipates that new experiences of yogurt will not be "enjoyable," but positions the acquisition of a yogurt-based diet as supplemental to a milk-based one: if one is already following Davis's recommendation that milk replace water, the wholesale shift to yogurt marks an embrace of the potential of the microbial to alter the body from within. Invoking an industrial metaphor of the body's mechanical use of these yogurt-provided allies, she writes: "Yogurt bacteria synthesize, or make, the entire group of B vitamins in amounts sufficient for both themselves and their host; thus the person who uses yogurt liberally has a 'B-vitamin factory' in his intestines."[26] Davis has a fundamentally mechanical view of the body's operations, which grounds her understanding of taste: taste is merely a mechanical reaction that can be recoded through moral self-fashioning. In the following, the problems of the mechanical functioning of the body is discussed in terms of "tolerance," a view of the colony within and its ability to accommodate the microbial visitors that food brings with it. In a paean to the autointoxicating putrefaction of Kellogg's conception of rotting from within, Davis writes:

> If digestion is below par, the protein and calcium from yogurt are more available to the body than are these substances in sweet milk. . . . The yogurt bacteria living in the intestines break down milk sugar into lactic acid; since the bacteria which cause gas and putrefaction cannot live in lactic acid, they are largely destroyed. It is for these reasons that persons suffering from digestive disturbances or milk allergies can usually tolerate yogurt without difficulty; and that yogurt is especially valuable to use as a formula for sick infants.[27]

In yogurt, Davis finds a primordial foodstuff, a panacea that can serve as food for babies and be easily digested by those who have developed intolerances for specific foods. Yogurt also has the potential to restore health, serving as a means to make digestion possible in ways that have been lost through a wayward diet. Her underlying logic of substitution—that water should be replaced with milk, and that milk can be replaced by yogurt in times of ill health—suggests that an embrace of the microbial provides a means to reunite with nature through diet. Yogurt is one of the means this can be achieved through, but being able to consume yogurt depends on the cultivation of one's taste for it.

In the following, Davis offers her clearest appreciation for the microbial and the wars that are being waged within the body through modern medicine, which diet can counteract. As a synthesis of her thought, it brings together her understandings of what is happening in the body, mechanically, as it interacts with the components of the food one eats, on the one side, with the broader social context of eating in the United States, on the other. That context is one in which medicine is disrupting the body's natural processes and in which Americans have lost a taste for foods that might serve to restore health.

> It appears that [the valuable bacteria that produce B vitamins] grow best on milk sugar and cannot grow unless fat is supplied them; milk-free and/or fat-free diets, therefore, may be dangerous. The taking of sulfonamides and antibiotics, such as streptomycin and aureomycin, completely destroys these valuable bacteria; symptoms of multiple B-vitamin deficiencies may quickly appear unless food which promotes the growth of desirable intestinal bacteria, such as yogurt, is eaten. This food, sometimes spoken of in America as a fad, has been eaten for centuries in countries from Turkey to Lapland, Iceland to China. A study . . . points out that when yogurt is eaten over a long period, no other bacteria except those from yogurt are found in the stools.[28]

Yogurt is portrayed as having a permanent effect on the individual's body, the results of which can be demonstrated in the microbial excretions made by the body; from within, the yogurt cultures transform a body's ability to digest in ways that are "found in the stools," a form of evidence that makes evident the bodily interior and its operations in ways that are otherwise invisible. The challenge, however, is that yogurt is a recurrent "fad" for American consumers and depends on Davis's appeal to its historical and global ubiquity to defray anxieties about its strangeness. And in her global appeal ("from Turkey to Lapland, Iceland to China"), Davis brings together the whiteness of Europe, portrayed in the whiteness of Finns and Icelanders, with the racially coded people of southeastern Europe and China; as a multicultural appeal, it relies on readers finding the strange increasingly familiar through the proximity she produces in an appeal to Europe. That rhetorical work is manifest in the Colombosian family's introduction of yogurt to American consumers and the paths to popularity yogurt was plotted on in the mid- and late twentieth century.

## Making American Yogurt

Histories of yogurt tend to retell the same story of accidental discovery, coupled with its consumption as based in necessity brought on by environmental hardship, as if yogurt is intrinsically unappealing and only desperation would lead a person to consume the curdled liquid that an early yogurt might present itself as without the purifying effects of industrial processing. For example, introducing his Armenian American wife's cookbook, *The Book of Yogurt,* David Kaiserman introduces himself through his seemingly typical experience with yogurt as a food in the American twentieth century. "My initial encounter with yogurt as a ten-year-old was negative enough for me to dismiss it at once and rush back to my favorite all-American dairy products, milk and ice cream. In time, . . . I came to know and appreciate many different cuisines from around the world. . . . As for yogurt, it simply never entered my mind to try it again."[29] That is, until he met Sonia Uvezian, who introduces him to the pleasures of yogurt through her cooking. As he seeks to introduce yogurt to an American cooking public, he tells a version of the repeated story of yogurt's origins, mingling fear of becoming "sick" with a sense of "desperation":

> [Yogurt] is generally considered to have originated in the Middle East in what is now Turkey or, perhaps, neighboring Iran. Several theories have been advanced as to how yogurt was first created. One widely held theory is that a desert nomad, setting out on a journey, put some milk instead of water into a goatskin bag, which he then slung over the back of his camel. The heat of the sun and the bacteria in the bag combined to curdle the milk and transform it into yogurt, much to the nomad's astonishment when, hours later, he opened the bag to quench his thirst. Understandably frustrated (and probably desperate), he took a chance and tasted the custardlike substance, found it pleasantly tart and creamy. Later, still alive and not even sick from the experience, he shared his discovery with his fellow tribesmen.[30]

Kaiserman ascribes "astonishment," "frustration," and "desperation" to his "desert nomad," which casts his discovery as something that happens by accident. He also imagines the experience of taste, casting it as "pleasantly tart and creamy." This is implicitly positioned to counteract the presumed disgust his desert nomad was experiencing after finding that his milk has transformed into acrid yogurt through a chemical process that Kaiserman can understand in retrospect but was seemingly impossible to know in the moment of creation. It is a tale of discovery that traffics in an Orientalist racism that denies ancient people a possibility of intelligence in their actions, ascribing it instead to pure luck. Equally, yogurt's invention may have occurred through deliberate experimentation, the result of careful observation, but positioning it as an accident aligns it with unadulterated nature, a product of natural happenstance that could occur to anyone, and presumably has occurred countless times without purposeful human intervention.

Yogurt's invention may also have occurred in the house, which Kaiserman suggests in an alternative tale of yogurt's origin story, this time relying on a form of primordialism that places yogurt's beginnings in prehistory:

> Another theory places the original discovery of yogurt at an even earlier time than that of the nomad, somewhere around the dawning of the Neolithic Age (about 10,000 B.C.), when man first learned about milking. A clay pot filled with milk was left outside, perhaps inadvertently, for several hours, with the result that the milk turned into yogurt. The combination of the hot climate of the Middle East and the absence of sanitary conditions provided a fertile environment for the yogurt bacilli to exist naturally and to multiply.[31]

Again, yogurt is accidentally discovered and this time it is as a result of poor "sanitary conditions." What those sanitary conditions were is left to the reader's imagination: could the same pot have been used as a chamber pot, or was it merely used for handling the viscera of prey, whose microbial colonies were left unwashed from the pot before its use for storing milk? In both cases, yogurt is a happy discovery and one that the communities who stumble on it continue to reproduce, ignorant of the microbial nature of their discovery. Presumably their interest in yogurt is based entirely on its "pleasantly tart and creamy" taste, one they need little cultivation to appreciate given the "desperation" of their times.

Yogurt's unclear origins also led to nationalist claims based on growing understandings of the microbial nature of the food and its geographical associations. Yogurt is the product of two distinct microbial lines, *Bacillus bulgaricus* and *Streptococcus thermophilus*. The former was first isolated by Bulgarian scientist Stamen Grigorov in 1905 through examination of a sample of yogurt from Bulgaria.[32] Further research has shown that it is a naturally occurring microbial culture in the plants of the region and in the intestines of local herbivores.[33] *Bacillus bulgaricus* ties yogurts together through time, suggesting that anyone who has eaten yogurt has participated in the consumption of a microbial colony that any human can potentially share. Its geographic specificity might also lend itself toward an origin story, but in its absolute unknowability, nationalist claims attempt to provide a narrative of superiority, if not certainty. In his voluminous history of food, *The Foodbook,* James Trager recounts:

> Bulgarians claim that only the mountains of their country can produce the *Bacillus bulgaricus,* and that only this bacillus can curdle milk the right way for good yogurt. They say, too, that the milk must properly be goats' milk and water buffalo milk, a brew twice as rich in butterfat as cows' milk. Bulgarians eat as much as six pounds of yogurt a day and claim that yogurt made elsewhere is a disgrace.[34]

Six pounds of daily yogurt exceeds Davis's comparatively modest four cups to be consumed in times of illness, but Trager is echoing a curiosity with yogurt and its medicinal properties that Ilya Metchnikoff inaugurated by attempting to explain the longevity of Bulgarians in the early twentieth century.[35] Interested in Bulgarian diets, Metchnikoff isolated yogurt consumption as the likely route to longevity, itself based on his understanding of the potentials of microbial consumption. This would later be picked up in Gayelord Hauser's *Look Younger, Live Longer*[36]—itself a direct inspiration for Davis's dietary recommendations—and resonated elsewhere, including in Maguelonne Toussaint-Samat's *History of Food,* where she writes in appreciation of yogurt's medicinal properties: "Lactic acid, if not absolutely guaranteed to make you a centenarian, is very good for the digestive system, except in a few rare cases of allergy to milk. It destroys the microbes causing putrefaction (which is not digestion but its opposite), which are present in intestinal infections and cannot live in an acid environment."[37] Like Kellogg before her, Toussaint-Samat relies on the putrefaction-fighting powers of lactobaccilus to explain the powers of yogurt and its appeal, as if it could not simply be something that people have a taste for eating.

Whatever its actual origins, yogurt was commercially introduced to the United States in 1929 by the Colombosian family of Massachusetts. Across the archival material available (newspaper articles, magazine profiles, trade journals, and internal documents), the details vary slightly, but the story is consistent, even if the dates shift. Starting in Andover, outside of Boston, and eventually relocating to Metheun, Rose and Sarkis Colombosian began by making and selling small batches of yogurt made from excess milk produced at their family dairy, reportedly using a strain of bacillus that Rose brought with her when she emigrated from Turkey during the Armenian Genocide. Sarkis had arrived in 1917, with Rose moving to the country in 1922 after the death of her first husband; they met through a friend and were eventually married, having two boys, Joseph and Robert (Bob), in the years to come. In the beginning, Rose helped to support their family by selling their niche product, plain yogurt, to other Armenians in the greater Boston area, which Sarkis delivered; Rose worked in the home, preparing the yogurt on the stove, and Sarkis served as the public face of the endeavor, slowly extending their market reach throughout the Northeast. Bob Colombosian, who inherited the business from his parents, recalls this period: "My parents were Armenian. Mother knew how to make cheese and yogurt on the stove. So she started making yogurt from our extra milk and we would hand deliver it in the local area— maybe a dozen quarts or so. In the early 1930s, word was getting around. Yogurt wasn't known among the Yankees, but my father would drive into Boston in a car that had been made into a truck to sell the yogurt to ethnic food stores."[38] Over time, their product began being distributed to grocers who served communities drawn from throughout the Middle East and southern Europe, making its way into small "ethnic" grocery stores; by the 1960s, they were distributing to health food stores as well. By the 1950s, they had capital enough to invest in a small factory after a fire burned down their earlier production facility, and by the early 1970s, the new factory was successful enough to support the transition to a larger factory in Metheun. The transition to the factory in Metheun coincided with financial complications at local distributors that resulted in the selling of the company to a French cheese maker, Bongrain, in an effort to save the family's finances and the company. Thereafter, Bob served as a consultant, ran an experimental frozen yogurt stand, and was eventually enrolled in an advertising campaign for the brand that highlighted its ethnic roots and ties to New England. Eventually, Bongrain sold Colombo to General Mills, the American food conglomerate that makes Yoplait yogurt.

Until the 1970s, Colombo yogurt was available in one flavor: plain. Yogurt was a slowly growing market that relied in the first instance on increased migration to the United States from southeastern Europe and the Middle East, an effect of the growing industrial development in American cities and continued conflicts in the regions people migrated from. Bob recounts the period in the 1970s: "During the '40s, we used to fill glass yogurt containers by hand. Then, we went to an automatic process in the mid-'40s and filled about 2,000 quarts a week. By the 1960s, Colombo, Inc., was filling between 15,000 and 20,000 quarts a week."[39] In a story presented in the *Colombo Yogurt News* in 1973, the growth in the market is apparent:

> In 1971, Americans ate a whopping 100,000 tons of Yogurt, or roughly 200,000,000 pounds. And, the American Dairy Association says that people eat Yogurt not just to help in losing weight or to stay healthy, but simply because they like it. Traditionally, plain Yogurt is eaten in the Middle East as an integral part of the daily diet, and mixed with meats, fruits, and vegetables. During the 1950's in the United States, Yogurt manufacturers began adding fruits and fruit flavorings to plain Yogurt, enhancing the slight tang.

At once, this document points to the ethnic roots of yogurt, associating its plain presentation with its origins in the Middle East, while also pointing to how yogurt was actively adapted to the American market by "enhancing" the taste through the use of fruit and fruit flavorings. That "enhancement" runs parallel to the "cultivation" of taste, suggesting that the added fruits and sugars do not so much cover up or eradicate the "slight tang" as complement it so as to meet the tastes of its consumers through careful adulteration. In the business-focused *Griffin Report* in the mid-1970s, as the Colombosian brothers handed control of the company to Jim Wells, the market assessment is frank: "What makes one yogurt brand or product more attractive than another? . . . While price is sometimes a factor among certain users, it's basically taste and consistency that determine which items sell best. Interestingly enough, . . . people who start off with flavored yogurt often go back to plain yogurt once they get used to using the product regularly."[40] There is hope expressed by Wells that a consumer attracted to the healthy basis of yogurt but tempted by its flavors and sugars might be cultivated to experiment with plain yogurt; but "taste" looms over the decisions that consumer makes—not the apparent health benefits of yogurt, which are subject to the whims of passing fads.

Over the course of Colombo's history, market research conducted for the company provides insight into the American yogurt market, or at least the kinds of concerns that the Colombosian brothers brought to their management of the company. In 1976, as the Colombosians brought Wells in as president of the company, marking the company leaving family control, market research summarized in the *Griffin Report* shows that "the typical yogurt eater is a young clerical or professional worker in a big city between the ages of 18 and 28 with an expanding income potential. . . . [And] there are many other people who once they tried yogurt might become regular customers." Nearly a decade later, in a document prepared for Colombo customers around 1984, entitled *History of Colombo,* readers are told: "Colombo is the *original* Yogurt Dairy in America. . . . Originally, yogurt was consumed only by certain groups of people whose origin was Middle Eastern. Today, the perception of yogurt is a nutritious, natural food that is enjoyed by all groups of people." As an internal document prepared for a constituency based outside of Colombo's original territory, the investment in casting the original audience for yogurt in the Middle East situates the food as resolutely "ethnic," despite Armenia being in Europe. In the same document, as an explanation for how yogurt came to appeal to mainstream, white American consumers, the writer provides: "The addition of fruits and flavorings made the tart and tangy flavor of plain yogurt much more palatable for new yogurt eaters." This adulteration was critical in reshaping the taste of yogurt to meet the appetites of Standard American Diet eaters and grow the market of yogurt consumers.

Those "new yogurt eaters" were the ones adopting yogurt as a new food, a possibility enabled by its transition to something more palatable to American tastes by being sweet and fruity. In a description of current and growing demographics in an internal document, this is made plain: "Established: female; 18–49 years old; disposable income (above average); generally, better educated; nutrition oriented. New entries: children, men (fitness), older adults (health & diet)." If yogurt's main appeal before the 1980s was as a healthy food, and one relatively free of fat, Colombo sought to capitalize on that characterization, despite its increasing use of sugar and fruity flavors to make yogurt palatable for more Americans. "Fitness" and "health & diet" as drivers both point toward this; yogurt's way forward was as a "health and dietary" food, free of the dangers of junk food. As Bernice Kanner wrote in *New York* magazine:

> Yogurt's biggest lure is not its taste or even its snob standing (yogurt is, after all, considered a food for highbrows and cultured palates) but rather its purported health and dietary benefits. Yogurt contains a fraction of ice cream's fat and cholesterol. However, there's no definite link between it and longevity, though Dannon implied such a link years ago in its famous commercials about the centenarians in Soviet Georgia.[41]

She carries her geographic associations with health further:

> Greeks used yogurt to settle upset stomachs. Indians to regulate the intestinal tract. Americans got their initial taste of it in 1870, when Turkish immigrants brought some with them. The first commercial batch was produced here by Sarkis and Rose Colombosian; . . . by the mid-1930s they had begun supplying their Colombo brand to Greeks, Syrians, Armenians, and other ethnic Americans.[42]

Throughout, Kanner associates yogurt with health and with "ethnicity" of one form or another, ranging from Soviet Georgians to "ethnic Americans." These associations have been provided for her throughout the history of marketing yogurt to the American public, which regularly relied on shared qualities between yogurt and ethnic difference, in both internal documents and public-facing narratives. This reliance on ethnic difference and its association with nature is one the Colombosians accepted, particularly in relation to ideas about taste.

The research on the American market was necessary for Colombo's corporate efforts because, for many Americans, yogurt was a foreign substance. Recounting the early days of Colombo's entrance into its local market, Bob provides a reporter with the story of yogurt's fundamental misrecognition as not-food: "Spreading the gospel about yogurt wasn't always easy. To Armenian immigrants like the Colombosians, yogurt was familiar, a condiment you spread on everything from grape leaves to spicy food. But when [Bob] Colombosian first brought yogurt into Andover schoolhouses, some teachers mistook the snack for skin cream."[43] At least it likely did no harm to the teachers who smeared it on their body. But, as food, it was apparently suspicious to significant portions of the American population, as discussed in *New York* magazine in the 1980s, with dramatic differences in local consumption patterns. In assessing the American market for yogurt, Kanner wrote that, "according to Mediamark Research, . . . folks who live in St. Louis are so sour on yogurt that they're 25 percent less likely to eat it than the average American, and, for unknown reasons, less than half as likely to touch the stuff as the average San Franciscan."[44] Given yogurt's association with natural food and its punny association with being "sour," it is no surprise that, in the 1980s, it would be adopted in California's growing health cultures and neglected elsewhere.[45] Kanner allows the comparison to be underdeveloped, though, suggesting that the buying public of California might be more cosmopolitan in their tastes than that of St. Louis—or at least accepting of yogurt's "sourness." Elsewhere she explains:

> Make no mistake: Yogurt is still the smallest segment of this country's $33-billion dairy industry, and our consumption per capita is miniscule with that of Europeans. In 1980, the average American downed just 2.6 pounds (about 5 cups) of the stuff, while the average Frenchman polished off 40 cups, the average Dutchman 60 cups, and the average Swiss 200. Still, yogurt has been the fastest-growing part of the United States dairy business over the last decade.[46]

As a set of comparisons, the Californian consumer is more akin to the yogurt-devouring Swiss consumer, the St. Louis consumer dragging the American average downward. As much as the market may have changed over the years, by the mid-1980s it had not changed so much that yogurt was entirely mainstream, even with the sugars and fruits added to it to appeal to consumers of the Standard American Diet.

In a General Mills produced press release celebrating Colombo's seventy-fifth anniversary, a timeline is provided of Colombo's innovations. These include being the first to "develop mix for frozen yogurt" in 1968, the introduction of "Fruit on the Bottom Yogurt" in 1970, the

introduction of the "first non-fat plain yogurt" in 1977, and the reintroduction of full fat plain yogurt in 1991. It also claims Colombo as "the
No. 1 plain yogurt company in America, with sales exceeding $8 million"
in 1976. This is the same year that Bongrain acquired Colombo, coinci-
dent with its market peak; in 1993, General Mills acquired Colombo,
first preserving it as a regional brand, and eventually discontinuing it in
2010. In the same flyer, General Mills provides updated market information on yogurt's consumption, claiming: "Yogurt is a very popular food
item for Americans, with almost 75 percent of American adults eating it
and most eating it at least once a week." Beyond that, they write: "Eight
in 10 women eat yogurt, with 50 percent eating it at least once a week. Although men do not eat as much yogurt as women do, still, 63 percent say
they consume this tasty treat." In the seventy-five years of Colombo and
its market research, the breadth of who was consuming yogurt steadily
grew, as did their reasons for eating it; they successfully charted the course
from an ethnic, fringe food with a limited audience to the American
mainstream.[47]

During the same anniversary year of 2004, Bob was interviewed for
the local North Andover newspaper, the *Eagle-Tribune*. In his old age,
now separated from the company and brand by several years, he was forth-
right in his feelings about what had happened over the course of Colombo's history, particularly the attempts to appeal to American tastes: "The
American public loves sugar. If they could eat it without the yogurt, they
would."[48] Bob goes on: "Today the stuff you get isn't even yogurt. Once
you started adding sugar, I don't know what it is anymore."[49] Yogurt, for
Bob Colombosian, is only really yogurt when it is in its natural state, tart
and plain; but the currents of American consumerism pushed yogurt
away from these qualities and toward sweeter and more palatable flavors
for mainstream consumers. Throughout their market research, strawberry
flavoring consistently ranked the highest among American consumers, a
combination of sweet and fruity that chafed against Bob's sense of purity.
The best epigraph for Colombo's story might come from Wells, when he
was interviewed for the *Griffin Report* in 1975: "We're in a fast-moving
business and only those who can respond quickly to consumer tastes and
product variations can make out in it. Only those companies who understand that we're basically in a cultured product business will, in the

long run, be successful in it."[50] At heart, Wells accepted that the reality of selling yogurt was in accepting its natural "tang" or tartness as a "cultured product;" there is only so much that can be done with the taste and only so much the standard American palate can bear. Those tastes might be shaped through appeals to health, as Davis attempts to achieve; they might also be modified for good or ill through appeals to yogurt's ethnic roots. Ultimately, Wells suggests that consumers either have the taste for yogurt or they do not. Colombo made yogurt as "white" as they could, adulterating it in ways that Bob objected to aesthetically but accepted commercially. In the end, that was not enough to save Colombo as a brand. Instead, the shelves are now full of sugary and fruity yogurts, the plain varieties tucked in among flavors that seek to "enhance" yogurt's natural properties.

## Our Common Microbial Kinship

As both a token of the natural-foods movement in the United States, and a microbial supplement, yogurt provides a way into the shifting currents in the Standard American Diet in the twentieth century. From something resolutely "ethnic" to something ubiquitous in grocery stores and on menus, yogurt charts the uneasy but steady acceptance of microbial foods through popular appeal, as health food, and through adulteration. As a form of medicine, it is meant to be palatable, something that one can eat regularly to ensure good health, but also, as Davis suggests, something that one might consume in large quantities in times of physical distress. Like Kellogg's use of yogurt-based enemas, the mass consumption of yogurt provides a suggestion of how yogurt was conceptualized as medicine, potentially more so than as food in the strict sense, as a means to popularize it for American consumers. Its edibility was secondary to its uses as a health supplement or medicine, until it could be shaped to meet the expectations of American eaters, which meant that it needed to be "enhanced" to the degree that its nature was held in check by the sugars and fruits that companies added to make it palatable to many Americans.

While working on this chapter, I admit to having consumed a significant amount of yogurt. Reading and writing about it kept it at the forefront of my awareness, and I found myself considering the history of the stuff as I sat down with a bowl of yogurt, which was slightly adulterated with maple syrup or honey, or heavily modified with coffee or vanilla flavoring. The market for yogurt, healthy or not, has expanded to a degree that the Colombosians could probably not have imagined a century ago, and while plain yogurt is a staple in our house, I find it buried at the end of a supermarket aisle, past all of the mainstream yogurts and nestled in a collection of natural foods, high-end imported yogurts, and yogurts made with other forms of milk than simply cow's—but not water buffalo. The successes that yogurt has had as an everyday foodstuff have been predicated on its adaptability and the cultivation of an American market that accepts the "tang" of the product alongside its fruity "enhancements."

In writing about the history of Colombo yogurt, I found myself longing to try a food I could never taste. If I ever ate Colombo yogurt in my life, it is not a taste I remember, and I longed for the visceral connection to the history of a family I would also never know. I find the possibility that all American yogurts descend from the strain of *Bacillus bulgaricus* that Rose Colombosian brought with her to the United States in the early 1900s a tempting story; that American consumers of yogurt share a common microbial colony, a common somatic incorporation, even if it has slightly changed over time, is a tempting fantasy. Its temptations lie in the historical connections that yogurt might make material: a microbial connection exceeds something more arbitrary like "tradition." Instead, a connection through yogurt offers a kind of kinship through shared substance. Whereas this material history and shared connection might be benign, it is the inverse of the fears that have become associated with fecal microbial transplantation. Both share an interest in changing what is happening inside the body through what is introduced to the body from the outside, but microbial medicine in the form of food is largely accepted as benign: the most one must overcome is a sense of trepidation and disgust with specific foods. But fecal microbial transplants exacerbate these feelings and rely on desperation to ease one through their feelings of disgust. Before I turn to fecal microbial transplants, though, there is one last visit to make to our bodily interiors, through child-rearing and attention to what comes out of the body as a means to understand what is happening in a body and the makings and remakings of American disgust.

# Threshold 2
## TASTING WHITENESS

WHERE DOES DISLIKE BLEED INTO DISGUST? That's the question I wrestle with in working through my relationship to Rob Greenfield and his project of living on four dollars per day in a predominantly Black and poor neighborhood in the Atlanta region. I came across Greenfield's project while searching for food-desert interventions focused on probiotics; I wondered whether the recent turn toward probiotics had a profound enough impact on the American social imaginary that it had begun to shape how remedies for food deserts were being developed and implemented. Greenfield's blog turned up high in my search results. I hadn't known of him before—I don't think I'm his target audience—but he represents a kind of approach to American solutionism that is deeply familiar.

Greenfield is a self-described "dude making a difference." He characterizes his young adult life as typically American: he was "focused on money, nice possessions and the pursuit of women." At the age of twenty-four, he had an environmental epiphany and turned his back on his dream of being a millionaire by the age of thirty. He committed to living simply and drawing attention to the possibilities of anticonsumerist, low-impact living through a series of public-facing projects. He rode across the United States three times on a "bamboo bicycle," trekked from Rio de Janeiro to Panama while relying on the kindness of strangers, which became the basis for a documentary series, "Free Ride," and lived in a "tiny home" in San Diego, where he "grew a little of his own food, lived purely on rain water (approximately two gallons per day), harnessed energy from the sun using solar panels, created near zero waste and composted humanure." He then embarked on a month-long project to consume "like the average US American for one month and wore all the trash he created,"[1] which resulted in a costume composed of clear trash bags filled with his garbage. That resulted in a series of TED talks where he adorned the costume to admonish his audiences for their consumerist ways and offer hope for a less consumption-focused lifestyle. After that, he decamped to Bankhead, Georgia, to test whether one could live on the four dollars per day that is provided by federal SNAP benefits in the United States, a form of subvention to the poorest Americans to support their food expenses.

Why do I dislike this kind of project? Fundamentally, though Greenfield might cast the effort as a progressive one in that it attempts to address excesses and inadequacies of the American diet and their impact on the environment, it is a conservative project that aligns with the erosion of the social safety net that Republicans have pursued in the United States since the 1980s. Demonstrating that people can live on the meager funds provided by the federal government, even in the context of a food desert, erodes the ability to argue for greater benefits to the people that need them the most. Rather than helping the people he seeks to, Greenfield adds to their marginalization. To make matters worse, in demonstrating that people can live on the threadbare support provided by the U.S. government, Greenfield imposes his dietary desires on them, rather than learning from them about their foodways. Greenfield's activism amounts to a form of neoconservative neocolonialism, the imposition and justification of austerity politics and white, elite foodways on poor and marginalized Americans. I dislike it; it's disgusting.

Greenfield describes the project as an effort to help people "take back their health."[2] This is motivated by his understanding that Bankhead qualifies as a food desert, a federal designation that the U.S. Department of Agriculture defines as having the following qualities: "Accessibility to sources of healthy food, as measured by distance to a store or by the number of stores in an area; Individual-level resources that may affect accessibility, such as family income or vehicle availability; and Neighborhood-level indicators of resources, such as the average income of the neighborhood and the availability of public transportation."[3] Food deserts tend to occur in urban and rural spaces where access to healthy food is low, distance to grocery stores is far, and individuals lack the resources to be able to buy the healthiest foods. Food deserts are often the product of investment on the part of store owners, as many choose not to open stores in places that they associate with high levels of crime, low quantities of consumers, and low-income communities. In this way, food deserts are the byproduct of long-standing racist assumptions about urban spaces and classist assumptions about rural spaces; they are also the byproduct of a failure of the state to support consumers through SNAP benefits and store owners through aid for locating stores in low-density or low-income communities. Food deserts also produce parasites like Greenfield, who take advantage of racist and classist stereotypes about food deserts to pursue activist projects like his attempt to live on four dollars per day.

At the outset, Greenfield understands his project as targeted at nonwhite people, aiming to teach them a kind of financial acuity that he presumes they lack. He writes: "Bankhead is over 80% black people and when I looked it up I found a source that says it's over 90%."[4] This dovetails with his sense of danger, which appears throughout his accounts of his month of living in Bankhead. At one point, while he and his girlfriend were doing laundry at a local laundromat, he asked one of his fellow laundromat users where he might find some fresh produce, a recurrent concern of his, and she pointed him to a store in the neighborhood. As he left, "another woman made sure to tell me to be careful. A guy had been shot in the face two nights ago in front of a nearby store. He died in the ambulance. Another guy had been shot in the arm and leg just a few nights before. They didn't know why."[5] Elsewhere, he writes that he and his girlfriend left a social engagement so that "we could make sure we were home before dark."[6] These fears exist in tension with what is otherwise warm and supportive interactions with the members of the Bankhead community. The greatest threat he and his girlfriend faced were rats in the home they borrow from a friend.

Greenfield's greater sense of urgency is the diets he imagines the people of Bankhead to have. In another interaction where he asked a worker at a local market where to "get fresh produce," she told him to "take Uber to Publix." Another "man stocking the shelves really didn't know. In a confused tone his response was, 'like apples and oranges?' For the most part people are fairly boggled by the question of where to get fresh fruits and veggies but plenty of them do come up with an answer after some pondering."[7] Greenfield takes the "pondering" of this latter worker as evidence that he doesn't understand what "fresh produce" is, inferring that he doesn't eat it, when it is equally likely that he's flummoxed that anyone would need to ask the question, given that there are only two local stores where people shop for fresh produce, Walmart and Publix. Greenfield's naïveté is masked by his racist assumption about other people's diets. This is echoed by other people he interacts with, as in the following vignette he provides for his reader:

> When I was on my way out of the front door I noticed a couple ba-nanas at the checkout counter so I decided to ask the attendant be-hind the bullet proof glass window some questions. The bananas were 2 for $1 which is at least twice the price at a grocery store and he said he bought them at Sam's Club. I asked if people actually buy them and he said, "They do now. They didn't before I started telling people that it is healthy to eat fruit everyday." It was sort of ironic that he was talking to people about eating healthy food yet running a store with almost nothing but junk food. I asked if his customers eat any healthy food and he said, "Nothing but junk food." He lives outside the community and said he eats healthy at home. He said there's not really anything healthy to eat around here.[8]

Greenfield cannily casts his quest to promote healthy living on the con-straints of SNAP benefits as a project shared by this shop owner, who has taken it upon himself to import, and marketize, bananas from the local Sam's Club. Like Greenfield, he seeks to spread the gospel of "eat[ing] fruit everyday" at the cost of "at least twice the price" of what he paid for the bananas. Moreover, like Greenfield, he "lives outside the community" and commutes into Bankhead as a commercial venture. He differs from Greenfield in that he has an ongoing commitment to Bankhead and his fi-nancial benefit is qualitatively different from Greenfield's, which is largely reputation building, but they share a disdain for the people of Bankhead, captured in the shop owner's claim that they eat "nothing but junk food," which Greenfield uncritically reiterates. Their shared contempt for the people of Bankhead facilitates their parallel attempts to talk "to people about eating healthy food" and failure to address the systemic problems that make the community a food desert.

Greenfield is aware that people might criticize his efforts as pros-elytizing a lifestyle that is unattainable for the people of Bankhead, which he preempts by positioning himself as "not telling anyone . . . what to do."

> I am creating tools for people who want to eat healthy and could use the inspiration, information, and motivation to do so. I want to break the myths that prevent people from eating healthy. I know that there are massive barriers standing in the way for many people but I believe the greatest barrier plaguing the people of the USA is the myths and preconceived notions surrounding food.[9]

With his understanding that he is simply trying to pierce people's "preconceived notions surrounding food," Greenfield suggests that a more strictly economistic approach to eating is a vital one to adopt. To that end, he argues that "cost per calorie is one of the most logical ways of understanding what I can and can't afford for many of the foods I'm looking at for the $4/day budget."[10] On the surface, this might be a reasonable approach to planning a diet. But calories are a fraught concept, and not all calories are counted the same, which is made evident in the photographs that Greenfield complements his blog posts with, all of which depict the food that he is purchasing from local stores. In many cases, what the images show are dried legumes, rice, and vegetables. There are no dairy proteins—no milk, cheese, butter, or eggs—and no meats. Moreover, there are no images of local staples that are part of Southern foodways, including cornmeal and collard greens. A vegan diet might be palatable to many of the members of the Bankhead community, but Greenfield does little to bridge his tastes with those of whom he seeks to help. Given Southern food traditions' indebtedness to frugal living, he could have started halfway to his goal. Is it too much to suggest that his whiteness obscured this possibility, his paternalism too entrenched to be able to conceive the lives of others?

Critical studies of race and racism often portray whiteness as an unmarked category;[11] it exists through its relationships with marked racial categories like Blackness and Indigeneity, which help to demonstrate what whiteness is not. If Blackness and Indigeneity are associated with a proximity to nature, then whiteness is, de facto, associated with civilization. But there is something even more slippery about whiteness, and that is how its lack of definitive qualities provides the basis for whiteness as a form of transparency.[12] By this, whiteness can serve as a container for other qualities, and presumably does not affect those qualities through intrinsic qualities associated with whiteness. This is how, as a cultivated capacity, whiteness can become a form of embodiment. This is also how Greenfield can pass his vegan diet off as neutral and unmarked. This is not to suggest that a racially coded body can become uncoded; a Black or Indigenous body cannot become a white one in a racist society, but a racially coded body can exhibit capacities that are associated with whiteness.[13] This conception of bodies and their capacities facilitates interest in "cultivation" as an intentional project, both as a form of self-care and through the careful governance of individuals and populations on the part of the state. Whatever differences may exist between John Harvey Kellogg and Adelle Davis, what they share is an interest in cultivating this transparent whiteness, a state in which the body is a vessel for the substances that move through it. Ideally for both of them, that movement is unobstructed and facilitated by the body's lack of defined qualities, leading to optimal "wellness." Greenfield enacts this whiteness in his occlusion of his tastes and practices as cultivated features of his person.

Microbial medicine is troubling to individuals and to biomedicine precisely because of the cultivated whiteness of bodies. If a body ideally has no features but only capacities, and one of those capacities is the transparent containment of a microbial colony, the risk is that the body can become the thing that it contains. The old saw "you are what you eat" takes on a different bite when the potential is that what you consume might be "dirt"—or the microbial waste of another body, with undetermined effects on a host. "Safe" microbes can be introduced to "safe" bodies, hence the growing success of a substance like yogurt as a consumer good and microbial treatment, but that "safety" is ideologically produced and not benign. Knowing whether or not something is actually safe relies on more than an individual's physiology or taste; it requires, additionally, an infrastructure to support the production, dissemination, and consumption of food, and the support for classifying food as safe and desirable in a consumer market. That can range from a caregiver and a community identifying something as food to a global distribution network and multinational corporate conglomerates, but in each case, it depends on a constructed intimacy between giver and recipient, between food-producer and food-consumer. Greenfield substitutes conservative politics and the unmarked whiteness of his diet for this intimacy.

Greenfield is also a symptom of contemporary food thinking in the United States, which positions certain kinds of foods and ways of eating as inherently more healthy than other practices. As a form of admonishment, it often positions white, upper-middle-class foodways—the New American Diet—as the right way to eat, with variance from it being unhealthy at best and life-threatening at worst. In that way, the New American Diet serves as a coercive tool that shames individuals without providing them with the means to change their access to the diet or aid in the development of a taste for the diet. Consider Greenfield's discussion of what makes food "fresh," which is a parenthetical during his first-day search for food in Bankhead at a Dollar Store.

> (By fresh I mean not in a can or frozen but of course not truly fresh as it would surely have been shipped from a huge farm in some far-off place). When I walked in I asked a man stocking the shelves if there was any fruits or veggies and he said no. I asked if they had any frozen veggies and the answer was also no. After a short conversation, he realized I was trying to find healthy food and he told me I'd have to look really hard to find that.[14]

"Fresh," for Greenfield, is obtainable only if one grows one's food; anything other than farming one's food involves a spatial and temporal division between where food is grown and where it is consumed. In this frame, freshness is a nearly-unobtainable quality, which can be mitigated by one's privilege and access, through either proximity to a garden or farmers market or sheer economic buying power.

Beyond these concerns of access, there is the question of taste. For Greenfield, his vegan version of the New American Diet provides a wealth of things to eat and ways of eating them. But for the people he is seeking to convince to resign themselves to his diet, his assumption is that they do not already have foodways that draw on brining and pickling techniques. In his paternalistic way, he goes to great length to explain the process and benefit of probiotics, imagining his audience's uneven knowledge of microbes and their place in the world.

This is probiotic sauerkraut, just as yogurt is a probiotic, except there is no culture that has to be bought and added because the cultures exist in the air. Every breath of air you've ever taken on Earth has yeast in it and this is what is used in the wild fermentation process. I'm sure you've heard of sourdough and that is the same concept. Fermenting foods both preserves vitamins and minerals but also creates new ones so by fermenting foods we can actually increase the value of what we purchase or grow. . . . The bottom line is fermentation makes food more nutritious and supports a healthy immune system. Even though you can buy it [sauerkraut] for really high prices at some stores it is in no way a food for the elite. Making it at home is one of the least expensive ways to eat truly healthy food and it can be done with or without a kitchen without a single fancy or expensive tool.[15]

This explanation comes in the wake of his enthusiasm about making homemade sauerkraut, accompanied by images of his girlfriend holding the jars of cabbage aloft; their enthusiasm for probiotics is palpable. In his economistic way, he stresses the frugality of home fermentation, emphasizing that "there is no culture that has to be bought" and that the value of food can be "increased" by creating new nutrients through the fermentation process. Here there is no mention of taste, with the presumption being an association with yogurt and people having "heard" of sourdough, neither of which would prepare the uninitiated to the taste of lactofermented sauerkraut. Despite all being processes of fermentation, how they occur and what their products are differ wildly. As part of the acquired palate of the New American Diet, they share associations, but for the uninitiated, they might offer some surprises that an appeal to frugality and value production won't ameliorate.

Beyond the question of taste are concerns with the safety of home fermentation. Greenfield brushes aside these concerns with an inelegant rhetorical association between his audience and "little kids."

Wild fermentation is not dangerous at all. The healthy bacteria and yeast that are supposed to be there create an environment where bad bacteria doesn't grow. . . . Know that it's easy and safe enough for a little kid to do and I don't know anyone who's ever gotten sick from fermenting their own foods.[16]

While there are some actual dangers in home canning and fermentation, largely associated with improper cleaning of canning jars, Greenfield dismisses them in two ways: first through an appeal to "wild" natural processes and second through his invocation of "little kids." In the case of the latter, the implication is that one needn't know too much to be able to make sauerkraut and need not have particular affinity for working with the necessary kitchen tools or ingredients. Is it too pointed to suggest that his paternalism borders on straightforwardly racist in his association of the people of Bankhead with "little kids"? Maybe so. In any case, his appeal to nature does similar work, establishing his audience as corrupted by civilization, not unlike Kellogg and Davis, captured elsewhere in his affective response to going to Walmart: "When I stepped into Walmart I felt a little sick to my stomach from the excessive materialism."[17] Civilization, Greenfield implies, creates a disgust response in him. That people could live in a way that he doesn't agree with or inspire empathy in him is affectively realized in his disgust. Greenfield may want to help the people of Bankhead and others living in food deserts, but he is uninterested in knowing them or why they live the lives they do.

Elsewhere, Greenfield recounts another occurrence of disgust, specifically in relation to eating uncommon foods. On his first grocery shopping trip in Bankhead mentioned above, he found his way into a Dollar Store where he finds a can of spinach. Adding it to a bowl of canned beets, rice, olive oil and salt, Greenfield explains:

> My reaction was "this is gross." I quickly gained one of my first understandings. A lot of people think vegetables taste gross and I've had a hard time understanding that. But this spinach was mushy and the beets were mostly void of flavor. I understand how people could think vegetables are nasty when this is their experience with vegetables. They don't even compare with the taste and quality of fresh vegetables, especially vegetables that are local and fresh. I haven't had canned vegetables in quite a while so this was a bit of an awakening for me.[18]

It's true that his lunch looks unappealing: he mixed the spinach into the rice and plopped sliced canned beets on top, seemingly straight from the can. A little finesse in the kitchen may have improved the results; what's possible with "local and fresh" produce demands technique and time when working with canned and frozen goods, which any chef will report. This is an additional "awakening" that Greenfield has during the course of his time in Bankhead, which he describes as affecting what makes "healthy eating" possible at all: "The barriers standing in the way such as accessibility, time, exhaustion, motivation, and education are probably stopping way more people in reality than money."[19] He recognizes that "time" serves as a barrier to people being able to take full advantage of their resources in a food desert.[20] And yet, he continues to come back to his view that "motivation" and "education" are equally important barriers, particularly in relation to "money." His solution, like so many white, "healthy eating" activists is to build community gardens, in seeming abeyance of admitting how much time, money, and motivation they require as well: "We are going to be building gardens for people in the community throughout the month so they'll be able to eat their own home grown veggies."[21] It's entirely predictable.

Is it too much to be disgusted at Greenfield's project, a straightforwardly paternalistic attempt to impose a different way of eating on a community in the name of "health," all the while supporting the neoconservative agenda of eroding the social safety net? Is it too much to dislike his disgust at other people's lifeways, their diets and consumerism? Maybe it's that Greenfield's politics are similar to my own but he takes the added step of intervening directly in people's lives and is willing to judge them without reflexive attention to his cultivated, affective responses, or that he lacks an awareness of the broader historical and political context of his project. More than anything else in his month-long account of living in Bankhead, I return to his reflection on walking through the abandoned neighborhoods of Bankhead: "It's a sad state to see so much go to waste and so many dreams crumble but there is a sense of beauty in seeing nature take back the land. The houses are growing over in trees and there is more green in this neighborhood than I've seen in many."[22] Greenfield's paean to suburban decay betrays his actual interests in a return of unfettered nature. If this civilization is corrupt, then let it return to nature. And, in the meantime, let them eat homemade sauerkraut!

# 4 The Arbitrary Rules of Disgust
## INTIMACY AND TOILET TRAINING

FAR FROM BEING UNADULTERATED REPRESENTATIVES of a primordial nature, children reflect a society's preoccupations with the body and behavior. Debates about the primacy of nature and nurture obscure that "biology" is always a mediating term between social forces and physiological capacities; biology and the body become sites where disgust and taste become located through somatic recompositions of the body and its capacities. But these reactive capacities are shaped purposefully, if often discretely, in order to create specific kinds of persons with critical sensibilities for the preservation of social norms. One context where this work can be appreciated is in the pages of parenting manuals, which seek to create a sense of what is natural and normal about children and parenting. In so doing, they promote social norms by creating guidelines for practice and expectations.[1] The market for parenting advice steadily grew over the twentieth century to become a massive industry in U.S. social life by the turn of the twenty-first century, in no small part due to the anxieties around childhood and expectations of "normal" child development. The influences of parenting advice run deep, in both negative and positive ways, and few advice-givers have had as profound of an impact on American parenting as pediatrician Benjamin Spock.[2] In his frequently republished *Baby and Child Care,* he describes the central importance of feeding in making a person:

> A baby girl (or boy) taking her first teaspoonful of solid food is quite funny and a little pathetic. She looks puzzled and disgusted. She wrinkles up her nose and forehead. You can't blame her. After all, the taste is new, the consistency is new, the spoon may be new. When she sucks on a nipple, the milk gets to the right place automatically.

She's had no training in catching hold of a lump of food with the front of her tongue and moving it back into her throat. She just clacks her tongue against the roof of her mouth, and most of the cereal gets squeezed back out onto her chin. You will have to shave it off her chin and scoop it back into her mouth. Again a lot will be oozed out frontward, but don't be discouraged—some goes down inside, too. Be patient until she is more experienced.[3]

Spock seeks to reassure the novice parent that their child's display of "disgust" is a reaction to the "newness" of the taste and consistency of the food they are being introduced to and the spoon used to convey it into the child's mouth—not a universal refusal of solid food based in some primordial capacity. Breastfeeding offers a foil, a situation in which the child exists in a "natural" relation with food and feeding. As one "shaves" the leaking cereal off the child's chin to reinsert it into the child's mouth, one may be battling one's own sense of disgust at the body leaking out what should be kept in. But such a reaction is as "trained" for the parent as eating solids needs to be for the child. That "training" is where social norms and cultural expectations of bodies become embodied. Parenting guides offer models of how embodiment becomes a practice, enrolling caregivers and children in projects that create children who reflect dominant expectations of behavior and personhood.

This chapter focuses on a set of problems associated with children and their digestion, from eating through excreting. What goes into a child and what comes out of that same child serves as the foundation for a set of everyday practices related to nutrition and health; they also serve as a diagnostic about what is happening inside of a child's body. Diarrhea or constipation are taken as indexes of something wrong in a child's physiological functioning or diet and can serve as a means to tinker with the child's food intake to ensure that they are healthy, often with assumptions about normal bowel movements and their regularity shaping these expectations of health. A child's diagnostic potential requires that the child's body is a neutral vessel, which requires, in turn, enculturation as a subject of a particular kind of cultivated disgust. Disgust serves as a control mechanism to ensure that what is going into and coming out of a child's body is what is expected; disgust serves to shape the body and its output in predictable ways so as to ensure that the excretory specimens that a body produces are transparent evidence of what is happening inside the body.

Caregiver intimacy is an embodied relation and is constructed through intersubjective conceptions of what occurs inside bodies, which taste can be a proxy for. This intimacy may respond to material cues such as the movement of bodies, gesture, and speech, but it is one that is fundamentally circumscribed by cultural norms and expectations about what the experience of intimacy should be. In the context of American sentiment, intimacy, like whiteness, is predicated on a conception of transparency, both to the self and to others.[4] Emotions are cast as plain, if not uncomplicated, allowing for a frictionless development of intimacy between caregiver and child, between kin, between lovers and friends. Practically, developing intimacy is much more difficult, and the wealth of parenting guides that seek to enable caregivers to create the conditions to facilitate the development of intimacy indexes just how difficult many caregivers accept the project to be.

It may seem strange that both parenting guides and medical procedures assume a transparent whiteness, an abstract blankness that can be acted on and responded to by an equally neutral and abstract actor, but both are the product of an American settler-colonial modernity that has sought to produce forms of whiteness that uphold and reinforce ideological projects that focus on normalcy and its aspirational qualities. Part of that normalcy is an unexceptionality that can be both desired and resisted. Being unexceptional means being unnoticed and without the need to be governed. Being unexceptional means fitting in. This provides the basis for diagnosis in that, when someone does not fit in to expected behaviors and social norms, it becomes obvious and can be acted on. Hence the parenting desire for a "normal" child, transparent in their affection and in their bodily functions. And so ableism and racism bundle together in the desire for a child who is a transparent container for the enculturation, care, food, and medicine they receive, known through their tastes and sense of disgust.

Here, I focus on a set of childrearing manuals, foremost among them Benjamin Spock's *Baby and Child Care,* which has steadily been in print in the United States since 1946, with regular updates. Spock's parenting is guided by the conviction that parents know more than they think they do and that "common sense" can inform sensitive and responsive parenting. For many American parents in the post–World War II period of intensive suburbanization and neolocality, Spock provided a seemingly ideology-free approach to parenting: he is committed to children first and foremost and provides a break from the psychoanalytically influenced parenting of the twentieth century, which often blamed parents for their children's abnormalities.[5] Spock's "common sense" parenting suggests that what he is presenting is based in a child's innate physiology and provides an understanding of human nature without adulteration and supported with adult supervision. The treatment of children, and especially babies and infants, serves as an aperture into American ideas about nature, particularly the belief that attending to what their bodies do and how they develop over time purports to demonstrate "natural" human development. But in reality, an examination of American parenting guides on nutrition, eating, and potty training shows how "human nature" is cultivated in specific ways to ensure that children's bodies remain "clean," which is a cleanliness that depends on an infrastructure of care that inculcates normative forms of disgust for parents and children alike. In the last section, I turn to "elimination communication," the practice of toilet training a child with limited or no use of diapers, as a way to conceptualize unsettling disgust. As a practice, elimination communication is rooted in an ideology of nature that a caregiver can build an intimacy to a child through anticipating their needs in ways that disrupt standard forms of regularity in American society. It also serves as a site to reconsider how natural one's disgust is at the functions of another person's body, providing the grounds for articulating a different affective response to the needs of other people.

## Taste, Diet, and Disgust: Sensibilities of Neutrality

As it did for Adelle Davis, milk provides a means into Benjamin Spock's conception of taste and disgust and their integral role in American social life. Milk is the primordial food for Spock, a resource that a mother can provide an infant, yet one that can be substituted through the use of non-human animal milk or formula with little effort and no detriment to the child. For Spock, a taste for one's mother's milk is inborn and acclimation to a new kind of milk can occur through careful exposure that is based in a child's curiosity, not forced feeding. The challenge that parents will face, as Spock outlines in the following, are the ebbs and flows of a child's taste for milk, which will alter as they incorporate other foods into their diet. Spock appeals to a crosscultural understanding that milk is universal, even if its sources may change based on local resources:

> Milk is a very valuable food. It provides good amounts of most of the elements that are important for a child's diet. . . . But it is helpful to remember that in the parts of the world where there are no cows or goats, children get these substances from other foods after their nursing period is over. It's also good to know that an average of a pint and a half (24 ounces) a day safely covers the needs of almost every child between 1 and 3 who is taking a reasonable diet otherwise. Many children between the ages of 1 and 2 want to cut down to this amount or less, at least temporarily. If parents worry and set to work to urge or force a larger amount, the children are apt to become steadily more disgusted. In the long run, they take less milk than if they had been let alone.[6]

For Spock, desire and disgust go together; the same substance a child can desire in one moment can become something they feel disgust toward in the next, based on its overuse or unwanted exposure. As it did for John Harvey Kellogg, disgust serves here as a means to regulate the body and its intake. If parents are too intent on a child eating something, whether the child likes it or not, the parent runs the risk of creating desire's opposite and a child's refusal to eat a "valued" food. Spock writes elsewhere: "The trouble is that children are also born with an instinct to get balky if pushed too hard, and an instinct to get disgusted with food that they've had unpleasant experiences with."[7] "Instinct" for Spock provides the foundation for refusal, in the form of "getting balky," but a deeper revulsion toward a food captured in his use of "disgust" is also possible to cultivate. Working with those instincts provides the framework for cultivating sensibilities that will ensure that what enters and leaves a child's body reflects the parents' interests.

Cultivating taste, for Spock, is based in a child's enjoyment of food. If an eating interaction becomes disciplinary, if parents insist that a child take "just a taste," they run the risk of spoiling a child's desire for a particular food and replacing it with disgust.

> I think it's a great mistake for the parent to insist that children who are feeding problems eat "just a taste" of a food they are suspicious of, as a matter of duty. If they have to eat anything that disgusts them, even slightly, it lessens the chance that they will ever change their mind and like it. And it lowers their enjoyment of mealtimes and their general appetite for all foods by one more degree.[8]

The risks that parents face in being demanding about food are both a specific disgust reaction to a particular food and a generalized loss of "enjoyment" in relation to the act of eating. Parents run the risk of turning their children into small Kelloggs, sapped of their passions for food and the "pleasures of the table." An infant's taste is largely indiscriminate: they will adapt to the foods in their environment, so the burden placed on parents, potentially, is to avoid reinforcing arbitrary eating practices that are less than ideal. As an example of this, Spock argues for the value of evaporated milk as a vital food for infants and children. When compared to pasteurized milk, Spock suggests, evaporated milk is sterile and "free of germs when you open it," "cheaper than fresh milk," can be "kept indefinitely," is "the same wherever you buy it," and is "a little easier to digest than fresh milk." He goes on: "When you have listed all these advantages, you wonder why anyone uses fresh milk. The main reasons are custom and taste. The taste of evaporated milk doesn't appeal to some older children and adults who have become accustomed to fresh milk. But babies love it, and they rarely object to changing back and forth."[9] Babies, Spock suggests, are indiscriminate in their love of evaporated milk; it is parents that are the problem, with their expectations of taste, which he implies are arbitrary. Doing what is best for baby is evident in Spock's discussion of introducing solid foods, in which he emphasizes the importance of children appreciating variety: "The exact order in which solids are introduced is not important. Cereal is commonly given first. The only disadvantage is that its taste doesn't have great appeal for many babies. Different babies prefer different ones. There is some advantage in getting a baby used to variety."[10] Taste, for Spock like for Adelle Davis, is a flexible and arbitrary capacity, but one that a parent can sour into disgust in their dogged insistence on particular foods that a child is resistant to eating.

The closest Spock comes to arguing that there is an intrinsic difference between one child and another is in his discussion of "overweight" children. His invocation of "constitutional" differences between children relies on his conception of differences between families, part of which is based on a difference in "taste."

> There are several factors that make for overweight [children], including heredity, temperament, appetite, happiness. If children come from a stocky line on both sides of the family, there is a greater chance of their being overweight. The placid child who takes little exercise has more food calories left over to store in the form of fat. The most important factor of all is appetite. The child who has a tremendous appetite that runs to rich foods like cake, cookies, and pastry is naturally going to be heavier than the child whose taste runs principally to vegetables and fruits and meats. But this only raises the question of why one child does crave large amounts of rich foods. We don't understand all the causes of this, but we recognize the children who seem to be born ("constitutionally") to be big eaters.[11]

One child has a taste for "rich foods like cake, cookies, and pastry," while another has a taste for "vegetables and fruits and meats"; one child is "placid" and takes little exercise and might come from a "stocky line." Spock's language indexes his understanding of how bodies desire food differently—he refers to it as "craving," a particularly visceral reaction—but it is not solely the desire for food that marks a difference in people. Some people, Spock recognizes, are born, "constitutionally," to be "big eaters," but what they crave are foods that are available to them in their social environment, which reinforce their tastes and appetites. This makes the difference between a "stocky" child and an "overweight" one. "Craving" and "disgust" are the two sides of appetite, one of which can be provoked through absence, the other through overexposure; both are the complex interactions of physiological capacities and social influences that produce them as everyday biological experiences.

The somatic basis of these reactions is apparent in Spock's discussion of disgust, appetite, and their interactions with illness. Sick children have a propensity to associate their feelings of illness with the environmental interactions they have during their illness, potentially symbolically contaminating otherwise benign foods with a sense that the food provokes symptoms of illness. Spock warns against caregivers "pushing" food on a sick child: "When food is pushed or forced onto a child who already feels nauseated because of illness, her disgust is built up more easily and rapidly than if she had a normal appetite to start with. She can acquire a long-lasting feeding problem in a few days' time."[12] While a caregiver might feel anxious about a child missing meals due to nausea, Spock suggests that forcing a child to eat while already feeling nauseated will likely result in an ongoing association between the food and the feeling, making apparent how fluid disgust is for children. Similarly, directly linking the emergence of disgust with a still-impaired appetite, Spock warns: "A very common time for feeding problems to begin is at the end of an illness. If an anxious parent begins pushing food before the appetite returns, it quickly increases the child's disgust."[13] What might be a fleeting symptom of an illness, albeit anxiety-provoking for a caregiver, can unfortunately turn into a longstanding form of disgust as the result of mismanagement of a child's appetite. In this way, an appetite based in natural curiosity and physiological need can be perverted, potentially leading to forms of disgust that can shape a person's life in ways that provide ongoing challenges. This echoes psychoanalytically informed approaches to childhood, but where psychoanalysis would accept disgust as a function of trauma wherein the symbolic association between an object and its source of disgust is relatively obscure to the disgusted individual,[14] for Spock the associations are plain: a food is directly associated with a period of illness and the experience of nausea. This association leads to an enduring sense of unease with a particular kind of food. The result is an arbitrary form of disgust that is based not on the intrinsic quality of a food, but on a set of accidental associations developed as a result of an untimely interaction.

Spock's discussions of bowel movements make the arbitrary rules of disgust plain. At once, he recognizes both that a child may be curious about what comes out of their bodies, and potentially even experience a sense of "pride," and that an "aversion" (i.e., disgust) can develop as a function of a child's growing desire for things to be "clean."

The positive pride in the movement, including its smell, and the enjoyment of messing in it if the opportunity arises are characteristic reactions of the earlier period [around 18 months] and can, in the latter half of the second year, be changed relatively easily into an aversion and a preference to be clean. I don't think it's wise or necessary to give a child a strong disgust reaction about his bowels or any other body function. But the readiness for a preference for cleanliness is part of what helps a child to become trained and stay trained.[15]

Rather than being intrinsically disgusting, Spock allows that excrement can be compelling to a small child, both the substance itself ("the enjoyment of messing in it") and the smell. Such an approach runs counter to assumptions about the excremental being innately abject or repellant; instead, it accepts that disgust as a reaction to bodily waste is something that must be cultivated. Moreover, Spock accepts the flexibility of a disgust reaction, allowing that there can be "strong" and, presumably, "weak" forms of the same instinct. A mild aversion to one's waste is necessary to stay clean, he suggests, but an overwhelming disgust reaction has the potential to lead to deeper psychological or social problems for an individual.

He discusses this psychological effect of abjection elsewhere, in an appraisal of the socially mandated need to be dirt-averse.

> Small children who are always sternly warned against getting their clothes dirty or making a mess, *and who take it to heart,* will be cramped. If they become really timid about dirt, it makes them too cautious in other ways also, and keeps them from developing into the free, warm, life-loving people they were meant to be.
>
> I don't mean to give the impression that you must always hold yourself back and let your children make any kind of mess that strikes their fancy. But when you do have to stop them, don't try and scare them or disgust them; just substitute something else a little more practical. If they want to make mud pies when they have their Sunday clothes on, have them change into old clothes first.[16]

Making a mess is something that children do, but they lack the sense of rules regarding cleanliness and dirt that animate adults and their social order. While children have a capacity for a generative form of disgust that can lead to upholding this social order—preserving order through a cleanliness Mary Douglas would recognize as managing danger and purity—this impulse must be cultivated carefully. The risk of disgust's mismanagement is the production of a "cramped" person, limited by their too-strong and overarching sense of disgust. Instead, through a logic of substitution, Spock suggests the use of more "practical" forms of mess-making: mud pies in a child's "Sunday clothes" might be too much for many parents, but changing a child into play clothes preserves their ability to make a mess while not leading to the development of an overweening sense of disgust and related social impairments. Thus, for Spock, while an interest in one's excrement might not be ideal socially, it can be modified over time to reflect broader interests in appropriate forms of mess-making.

Spock's view of disgust is an expansive one: rather than narrowly focused on substances that enter and leave the body, he understands it as a fundamental social reaction that guides everyday life. Like with children, it can be modified to appropriately reflect social norms and a sense of order. Reflecting on intergenerational conflicts around fashion, he writes: "Adults tend to be slower than youths in accepting new styles. What may horrify or disgust us one day may later become quite acceptable for ourselves as well as our children."[17] It is notable that Spock uses the same language to describe a middle-aged adult's reaction to bell-bottom pants and long hair on men as he does when he discusses a child playing with their own excrement. He uses "horrify" to capture the social unease and rejection of fashion trends to emphasize the register of disgust that such a banal element of everyday life can reach for adults; no similar verb is employed to consider a child's playing with their excrement or taking "pride" in its smell. As a flexible capacity, Spock casts disgust as serving as a means to somaticize distaste, thereby providing a visceral grounding for a moral order. Such an embodied reaction can be shared across a community, helping to constitute it as a community with a moral order founded in a common appreciation of dirt and cleanliness, but it resides in the individual and needs to be cultivated as such. Toilet training serves as a nexus for cultivating these sentiments in the context of a broader social order and the need to care for the self.

## What Goes In and When It Comes Out

Published by the U.S. Department of Labor's Children's Bureau in 1926, a guide to *Infant Care* implores parents: "Toilet training may be begun as early as the end of the first month. . . . The first essential in bowel training IS absolute regularity."[18] This call to regularity is a form of time-discipline, a means to inculcate a sense of self-regulation that aligns with the spatio-temporal organization of society as a whole.[19] As a form of time-discipline, ensuring that a child is having regular bowel movements works on both the parents and the child, governing how and what children are fed and when caregivers are to feed them. That it comes from the Department of Labor is no surprise: regulating bodies in these ways upholds normative structures of everyday life and its patterning, which regular bowel movements fit into, as do regular patterns of eating, sleep, and movement. As an imposition on nature, such regularity aims to align embodied experiences of nature (in this case, the need to excrete) with a desire for social order that scales between the infant's body, those of caregivers, and society as a whole, creating a hegemony grounded in claims about a foundational nature that has been created through social norms.[20] Natural forms of parenting, which Spock embraces, sometimes seek to counteract these norms in an effort to reach a truer relationship with nature. Writing against strict ideas about regularity, Spock notes:

> During the first half of this century, babies were usually kept on very strict, regular schedules. Doctors did not know for sure the cause of the serious intestinal infections that afflicted tens of thousands of babies yearly. It was believed that these infections were caused not only by the contamination of milk but also the wrong proportions in the formula **and** by the irregularity in feeding.
>
> Strict regularity worked well enough with a majority of babies. When they took an ample feeding at breast or bottle, it lasted them for **about** 4 hours just because that is the way a young baby's digestive system usually works.
>
> But there were always a few babies who had trouble adjusting to regularity in the first month or two—babies whose stomachs couldn't seem to hold 4 hours' worth of milk, babies who went to sleep halfway

through feedings, restless babies, colicky babies. They would cry miserably for shorter or longer periods each day, but their mothers and doctors dared not feed them (or even pick them up) off schedule.[21]

The regularity that the U.S. Department of Labor seeks to impose is an indiscriminate one; Spock's interest is, in the first instance, to nuance this form of time-discipline on the bodies of children and parents to allow for the idiosyncratic experiences of individual babies and their bodily capacities. A standardized schedule will always create friction with atypical bodies and for people and families that have irregular work schedules. But, in the second instance, Spock suggests that there is some truth to the schedule that the U.S. Department of Labor is putting forward, but that it is a coincidence with physiological functioning, which itself is dependent on the confluence of factors that shape what a baby eats, its experiences of eating, and its interactions with the people who feed it. In that respect, there is no "natural" schedule, but only one that accepts the complex social and physiological dynamics that undergird a baby's eating and excreting schedules and which comprise the biology of everyday life in a given society.

In response to the inadequacy of a standard schedule to shape the bodies and behaviors of everyone equally, the cultivation of habits serves as a means to create a sustainable pattern for individuals and families. Spock accepts that the basis of these habits must be a person's individual "patterns" and that these may or may not be "regular" in the way that the U.S. Department of Labor is invested in coordinating. Instead, habits allow for idiosyncratic schedules that provide individuals with a sense of control over their bodies; but ultimately, they need to be brought into accord with social patterns, from a family's schedule to society at large. He writes in praise of individual habits that:

> Everyone wants the child to turn out to be healthy in her habits and easy to live with. But each child herself wants to eat at sensible hours and later learn good table manners. Her bowels (as long as the movements don't become too hard) will move according to their own healthy patterns, which may or may not be regular; and when she's a lot older and wiser, you can show her where to sit to move them. She will develop her own pattern of sleep according to her own needs. In

all these habits she will sooner or later want to fit into the family's way of doing things, with only a minimum of guidance from you.[22]

Whether habits provide this structure or a standardized, regular schedule is imposed on an individual, the goal is the same: creating a body that is transparent and neutral in its activity so as to serve as a basis for knowing when something is wrong. An interruption to a body's regular bowel movements—diarrhea or constipation—provides a window into what is occurring inside of the body and also serves as a means to act against presumed disease. In this way, regular or habitual bowel movements provide a diagnostic tool to conceptualize the invisible interior of the body and to trace the influences that may have led to its disruption in sickness.

Diarrhea is often distinguished into "acute" and "chronic" forms in parenting manuals, with acute being associated with illness and chronic being the recognition that watery bowel movements are typical for small children. This is especially the case for breastfed children, who will often have softer and wetter bowel movements than their bottle-fed peers and older children who eat solid foods. Chronic diarrhea associated with a diet within the bounds of normal is to be expected, even if parents might find it undesirable to have to clean up and children find it uncomfortable. Chronic diarrhea might also serve as a means to isolate an element in a child's diet that they have an allergic reaction to or index stress related to social conditions, whereas acute diarrhea is a reaction to a virus or bacterial infection. As nutritionist Ellyn Satter explains in *Child of Mine,* her guide to pediatric nutrition:

> Babies and young children react to changes or distortions in their diets with more-frequent and watery stools. They often get diarrhea when they are teething, have a cold, or have a change in water or schedule. Antibiotics will cause diarrhea, probably because they disrupt the bacteria in the colon. At times, chronic diarrhea may develop following an acute bowel upset, although the child is no longer ill. Many times bowel habits return to their more-usual pattern once the stress has passed. Many times they do not.[23]

Satter goes on to suggest that, when compared to acute forms of diarrhea, "chronic, nonspecific diarrhea really presents more social and aesthetic problems than medical ones. Your general treatment of chronic diarrhea is somewhat diagnostic. By changing the diet you can find out what, if anything, is causing the loose and runny bowel movements, and, with any luck, get the stools to dry up a bit."[24] That Satter employs "social and aesthetic problems" to describe the challenge that chronic diarrhea poses for caregivers is an unlikely figuration, but indexes the disgust that she imagines many caregivers mingle with their anxiety about a child's health. What she seeks to do in alleviating caregivers' anxieties in this way is to attune sensibilities to the diagnostic potential of an irregular bowel movement, but doing so requires understanding the range of normalcy when it comes to a child's physiological functioning in relation to their diet and the social contexts that might lead to abnormal bowel functions.

As a way to introduce anxious caregivers to the normalcy of diarrhea in a child's life and the need for caregivers to react appropriately, Satter provides an anecdote of her overreaction to one of her children's seemingly abnormal bowel movements. Being reassured by her doctor that her child's bowel movements were "normal" served as reassurance for Satter and provided her with the basis for her understanding that chronic diarrhea is not something caregivers should worry about.

> Overreacting to changes in bowel habit can be simply asking for trouble. When our Kjerstin was six months old, her stools changed from their usual—a formed, even semi-solid, once-a-day pattern—to a three-times-daily pattern that was consistently softer and almost runny. I was concerned and thought there was something wrong with her. We happened to be at the doctor's office for a regular appointment, and I told the pediatrician that I thought she had diarrhea. She told me quite abruptly that it was not diarrhea, that it was simply a change in bowel habits, that my daughter was really quite normal and there was no cause for concern.[25]

Satter's use of "quite abruptly" indexes the frustration that her doctor felt regarding caregivers' concerns about diarrhea: from a clinical perspective, it is within the bounds of normalcy, yet caregivers become anxious about it in their hypervigilance about their child's health. Satter suggests that, if caregivers can approach diarrhea rationally, they can use it as a diagnostic tool. But this requires a form of intimacy with a child's bodily processes that may be uncomfortable for some caregivers, who choose, instead, to mask the physiological processes children's bodies undergo through diapering and reliance on expectations of independence that only older children can achieve. Ultimately, Satter seeks to reassure anxious caregivers: "Colons, like children, grow up. Some day you will no longer know your child's bowel habits in intimate detail."[26] The intimacy a caregiver develops in relation to a child's rhythms of eating and excreting serves as a means to know whether something is wrong inside a child's body and what might be done to correct it. In time, that intimacy erodes as a child is charged with self-care, with an acquired sense of the normal and abnormal in relation to rhythms and diet. One means some caregivers attempt to facilitate this maturation through is elimination communication, which depends on an intense intimacy between caregiver and child.

### Getting Back to Nature, Again: Elimination Communication and the Bourgeois Fantasy of Toileting

My introduction to elimination communication (EC), or "natural infant hygiene," was not to the practice itself, but to child-toileting in India, which serves as recurrent example for EC advocates. My partner and I were in Bhubaneshwar, Odisha, a place she had been traveling to for nearly twenty years at that point, first as a dance student interested in classical Indian dance forms and supported by a Fulbright fellowship, and more recently as a doctoral student in anthropology. She had deep connections there and stayed in a shared home that was frequented by international visitors (dance students, anthropologists, and other passersthrough). The home was run by a family who lived on-site in an adjoining private unit that opened onto a shared backyard, where they did laundry and cooked and their two children rambled.

One day, sitting outside, I observed the smallest of the children—who must have been two or three at the time—squat down, lift her dress, and poop on the cement back porch outside of the door to her family's home. She deposited a little turd on the porch and went indoors to wash up; her mother picked up a nearby hose, turned it on, and sprayed the little pile of shit into a nearby grate that opened into the sewer line, which carried the waste to an open-air sewer trough that ran behind the house and toward some distant processing center.

At the time, I don't think I considered what I had watched very deeply. I was continually stumped by the open-air sewage systems that I encountered throughout India, and this seemed like a continuation of that social system. It wasn't just the smell, a sensory distaste that I ascribed to my growing up in the United States, where our waste is hidden at all points; it was the routine flooding of the sewer systems that led to contaminated water and waterborne illnesses that really troubled me. It felt to me at the time like there was a widespread social acceptance of human waste, and I tried my best to inhabit an anthropological relativism, despite my sense that the open tolerance of human shit was also an invitation to chronic exposures to gastrointestinal illnesses, especially among the poor, who lacked ready access to filtered and treated municipal water.

Years later, after the birth of our first child, my partner and I were introduced to EC through the attachment-parenting books we read and my partner's involvement in the local breastfeeding community in Santa Cruz, California. We had already committed to using cloth diapers and EC offered the promise of a shorter time washing poopy diapers, which had its pragmatic appeals. No diaper changing is fun or desirable, and the occasional difficulty spraying off a flattened turd from a cloth diaper was a particular kind of chore. We bought a tiny potty but were uncommitted to EC as a parenting ideology; instead, we recognized that a bowel movement was likely to follow a meal and that getting our small child onto the potty after a meal often meant not having to clean a diaper.

As we became more aware of EC, we developed a sense of how it fit into a broader natural childrearing project that many of our peers subscribed to, which included EC, breastfeeding, unschooling, natural foods, and an obsession with communities that were accepted as living closer to nature, including people in India. Examples like the lived reality of our friends in Odisha were used to explain how being in tune with a child's bodily rhythms developed a sense of intimacy between caregiver and child, and that extended to a sense of an overarching natural order for human life that unsettled received conceptions of disgust. EC advocates claimed that diapers served as a convenience and mask of our relationship to this natural order, and EC and related practices offered an opportunity to get in touch with nature in a less mediated way. We had backed into many of these practices, in no small part because the surrounding community we were a part of reinforced them through a variety of discourses focused on the natural world, economic frugality, and environmental sustainability, but as anthropologists, we were both skeptical of the claims that EC brought anyone closer to nature, and the use of non-U.S. examples seemed to traffic in a form of neocolonial exoticism. For many parents we encountered outside of California, EC seemed a bridge too far, a kind of naïve naturalism that no parent would choose given access to cheap, disposable diapers. But as we watched our peers' infants grow into children with toilet anxieties, we felt sure that our early introduction of a potty eased our first child into a positive relationship with toileting.

In a representative discussion of EC in their *The Everything Guide to Potty Training*, Kim Bookout and Karen Williams lean heavily on EC's relationship with nature, suggesting that, through the cultivation of an attentive, EC-based toileting practice, a finer recognition of one's body and its capacities is possible.

> Elimination Communication (EC), also known as Infant Potty Training or Natural Infant Hygiene, is a natural, practical way to begin potty training far earlier than traditional toilet training techniques allow. EC can begin as early as birth or as late as parents are comfortable, but parents typically begin using EC between birth and four months. This is a clean, all natural way to teach your child from the beginning how to recognize and control his bodily functions.[27]

In three consecutive sentences, they invoke "nature" three times, associating it with EC's "practicality" and "cleanliness." EC relies on a caregiver's ability to attend to a child's needs in an immediate way, requiring the development of a sensibility that responds to individual patterns and is able to anticipate them in relation to basic conceptions of normal physiological functioning, such as putting a child on the potty after a meal in anticipation of the peristaltic action that is likely to result in a bowel movement. Such caregiving techniques are grounded in a sense for what is happening inside a child's body in a strictly physiological way.

But how "practical" EC is for many caregivers is questionable. Early on, it requires caregivers sensing and strategizing to ensure that children make it to the potty in time, which makes demands on caregivers and their attention. Since it is often supplemented with the use of diapers, the risks are only that a child will dirty a diaper if a toileting period is missed; yet, such misses might also be cast as a continued alienation from an intimacy with nature. In the following, Bookout and Williams work to make the stakes plain while continuing to lay emphasis on the natural basis of EC:

> Elimination Communication links to a timeless practice, still popular in Europe and Asia, where parents and caregivers learn to watch and listen to infants when it comes time to pee or poop. By focusing more directly on your baby's bathroom needs in much the same way you focus on your baby's nutrition needs, you can enable yourself to avoid common, everyday parenting issues such as fussy babies, dirty diapers, leaky diapers, and more. EC follows several simple steps to help parents and infants adapt naturally to what has always been a natural progression toward potty training.[28]

The appeal here to EC's global existence serves as a means to universalize the practice and isolate readers in the United States as the exception in their alienation from the natural process of learning how to toilet. The implication of this is that American parents have become inured to their children's "bathroom needs" in ways that are potentially harmful: the parallel Bookout and Williams construct with a need to pay attention to nutrition makes it plain that a child's health is at risk in a failure to attend to toileting in a responsive way. Yet Bookout and Williams attempt to make the appeal practical, emphasizing the ability to prevent "fussy babies, dirty diapers, leaky diapers." In so doing, they strike on two levels: first, an appeal to the practical caregiver who wants to avoid a fussy baby and changing dirty diapers, and second, a child's relationship to nature. The problem is that parents and caregivers must "learn to watch and listen" in ways that disposable diapers make redundant. Caregivers have to want a relationship with nature through the unsettling of their disgust; they have to want to know what is happening in their child's body in ways that are associated with conceptions of what is natural and normal; they need access to the resources of capital and time to make it possible as a counterpractice to regular time-discipline.

As an example of the dependency on capital to make natural parenting possible, consider attachment-parenting advocate and actress Mayim Bialik's narrative of her introduction to EC, which moves from a bourgeois disgust at the possibility of having to radically alter one's living space to accommodate the practice of EC to an acceptance that EC is part of a continuum of caregiving practices that share an affinity with natural approaches to parenting. In this way, EC is not out of bounds, but exists on one end of a spectrum of possible approaches to children, their bodies, and their waste, especially in the case of the fellow parent she meets, as she recounts:

> I met a woman through a mutual friend who was also pregnant. We got to talking, and she said she was having a stressful pregnancy because, upon deciding to practice "elimination communication" (also known as natural infant hygiene), she needed to pull up all of the carpets in her home before the baby arrived so that she would be ready on day one to start. That's not all. She went on to tell me that she was living in a tent in her backyard while this was being done. Very pregnant. In a tent. In her backyard. So that she could have a diaper-free baby. And her in-laws were questioning her sanity. Um . . . yeah, I was questioning her sanity, too! This new acquaintance and I ended up having our children on the exact same day, and we became very close friends in the coming months. Aside from my feeling that she was underhandedly trying to outdo my earthiness (aren't cloth diapers enough of an out-of-the-box statement?), she and I shared a lot of holistic and progressive philosophies and tendencies.[29]

Bialik's appeal to her fellow parent's sanity sets the stakes; it is not merely that EC is at the limit of what one might consider normal parental attention to a child's toileting, but that it requires a total reorganization of a family, which, given the context of American homes, requires substantial investment. In order to return to a closer experience of nature, as modeled by the Indian family we were neighbors with, Americans would need to invest capital in reorganizing their everyday lives, but potentially society as well, including broad support for non-diaper-based approaches to toileting. Bialik compares such an investment with her commitment to "earthiness," suggesting that part of the appeal of the use of cloth diapers is similarly a connection with nature, and also being "out of the box." Similarly, the use of reusable diapers requires upfront investment in diaper shells and inserts and ongoing costs associated with laundry and time to clean. Access to capital and time provide a means to get back to nature, to commit to unsettling one's disgust, and to break "out of the box" of American time-discipline.

In a YouTube video published in 2018 entitled "How to Never Use Diapers,"[30] Bialik provides viewers with an overview of her experiences with EC, which she eventually adopted with both of her children. Throughout the video, she emphasizes both the practicality of the decision to support her family's use of EC—namely, the reduction of diaper usage, the reliance on which she blames consumer capitalism for—and the intimacy that EC creates between a child and parent. She claims this intimacy as an experience that was "really, really powerful," yet suggests that

> EC is not for everyone. It is a big commitment in the first months, but it's not this exquisitely specialized or elitist practice. EC is practiced by women all over the world and before superabsorbent diapers were something that diaper companies told you that you needed, this is likely how your great-grandparents and beyond practiced pottying. What I found that EC did for me was it allowed me to cultivate the deepest level of intimacy with my children. I was able to meet all of their needs in a way that made sense to them and was comfortable for both of us. Especially for babies who are not verbal early on, which both of mine were not, this kind of communication was incredibly important.

Although Bialik barely mentions the global use of EC as a practice, commentators on the video focus their attention on the relationship between EC and communities outside of the United States. This focus exposes the deeply racist associations viewers have between the use of a practice like EC and the nonuse of diapers, which reflect dominant ideas about disgust. What is exposed in the comments is the politics of purity that continues to animate the use of diapers among many people and that motivates the continued refusal of a practice like EC, despite the claims that Bialik and other caregivers make about the intimacy built between caregiver and child. As an example of this, Donnalee Clubb responds to the video by writing: "I heard in India some people actually pee and poop in the streets, that a politician in that country actually ran on trying to get people to use toilets. So, [EC] seems gross." Clubb makes a significant leap between Bialik's reference to people practicing EC "all over the world" and the state of Indian politics; but this set of loose associations between toileting, dirt, and racial difference comes to the surface in relation to Bialik's benign claims about EC. Similarly, in response to the suggestion that wearing a diaper can lead to urinary tract infections and diaper rashes, Jennifer Webb writes: "'Possibly harmful to the babies health'? Um, these people [in India] literally shit in the WATER they drink from AND bathe in?? And now, India is releasing flesh eating turtles to rid the Ganges of the corpse problem . . . in their drinking water. With the awful stuff that is in their water, who knew diapers were just as 'harmful' lol?"

For these commentators, and for advocates of natural forms of child-rearing, places like India serve a vital symbolic role in the politics of purity. Because India is accepted as being less developed than the United States, it is also accepted as being closer to nature, a standard form of neocolonial racism. Similarly, parenting guides cast children, and infants especially, as being unadulterated and pure. It is through their enculturation that they move from being close to nature to being representatives of social norms and cultural expectations. Advocates and critics use non–North Atlantic places and people as ways to make claims about nature as pure and clean or dirty and dangerous, conceptions based in the same American logics of nature and purity. For some, nature is inherently pure, while for others it is inherently dirty. In both cases, it is a function of ideology that proximity to nature can be cast in these ways. Nature is always a project, subject to the politics of those who deploy it. The challenge here is that, when some children's bodies and the practices that guide their care are cast as being closer to nature than others, advocates also want to claim that they are closer to a state of purity—and, by extension, neutrality. In this, bodies and their functions are portrayed as being transparent in their processes, and that transparency provides the basis for caregivers to recognize whether a body is ill or healthy. But the functioning of a body or a person is never about the body alone, the functions of which are only partially based in physiology. Instead, the social forces and cultural expectations that a body is situated within and produced through shape its processes as a function of the biology of everyday life. Similarly, a person is shaped by the sociotechnical infrastructures that are available to that person; any individual body is representative of that infrastructure and its successes and failures. In this way, bodies scale. Bodies serve as an intermediary representative of social and environmental forces between the microbial and the societal and, in so doing, reflect ideologies about nature and its care. The microbiome is an example of this: what a person eats, what they are exposed to environmentally, and what their history includes are all potentially reflected in the colonies of microbes across and within a person's body. There is no clear causal evidence about what substances and exposures create and maintain which microbial colonies; nonetheless, it is apparent that our environments support the microbial life that, in turn, sustains human life. A too-sterile environment would kill off both our microbial life support and, in turn, human life.[31] Though hazy in causal relations, our microbiomes necessarily reflect our histories, and our social situatedness.

## Recomposing the Nature of Childhood

Focusing on children and childcare provides a means to demonstrate how society is reflected in individual bodies; children come to embody social norms and cultural expectations through their care, which is shaped, additionally, by the idiosyncratic beliefs and practices of caregivers and the physiological capacities of children and their social others. Together, this lays the foundation for the biology of everyday life—the ways that bodies are conceptualized, acted on, and created through ideas about the normal and abnormal, the natural and artificial.[32] In the context of social forms like industrial capitalism, diet becomes a central node for the exercise of expertise and practice. This leads to a focus on both what goes into a child's body and what comes out of it, the industrial production of appropriate foods and the societal promotion of toileting practices that are reflective of norms about bodies and presumed values related to regularity of bowel movements and where and how they take place. Parenting guides provide a means to track normative ideas about children and their natural states, from infancy onward, and how these natural states can be shaped by the caregivers in their lives with a focus on why appetites and bowel movements are sites of intense concern. Far from being a natural and transparent process, the social forces focused on children's eating and bowel movements demonstrate how experts attempt to make them natural and transparent, first through the desire to create "regular" bowel movements and tastes, and over time in the restoration of a more nature-based form of excretion and appetite. Appeals to nature and intimacy are grounded in an ideology of nature and purity that echoes interests in the transparency of whiteness, which is based in a natural restoration of individuals and society and their connections with the natural world. That conception of nature is necessarily produced through dominant ideas about bodies and their behaviors and caught in a recursive and reproductive logic that makes some bodies normal and others not. "Regularity" foregoes intimacy in favor of time-discipline and the imposition of a schedule on children's bodies.

Because of the construction of normal and abnormal bodies through the biology of everyday life, individual bodies are taken as metonymic representatives of a broader social order. A child who is "regular" is also a child who is normal, and a child who is irregular points to either a failure in their social shaping or an impairment of their physiological capacities. This representativeness of individual bodies is why there is such intense focus on the individual as healthy or sick and, by extension, what can be done to an individual body as a means to support its metonymic representation of a community. That an individual body bears this representativeness compels the governance of bodies on the part of those in power, whether they are parents, caregivers, health-care providers, or state actors. If part of providing care for a child is a focus on what goes into and leaves the body, such interest is an echo of the power that health-care workers have in the prescription of medicine and access to specific treatments, which is itself an echo of the power that states exert in the regulation of access to specific goods and treatments. In this respect, a focus on parenting guides provides an opening into the scalar operation of regulatory power, acting at all levels of human and nonhuman life in contemporary regulatory societies, with their interests in what can constitute life and the forms of life that are vital to society's reproduction. In the next chapter, I turn to the operation of state power and its regulation of fecal microbial transplants as a form of life-saving medicine and the state's interest in producing regularity as an iteration of state power, moving in scale from the care of children to the care of the body politic.

# Part II
## DISGUST AS MEDICINE

# 5 Normal, Regular, Standard
## THE COLONIZATION OF THE BODY THROUGH FECAL MICROBIAL TRANSPLANTS

CLOSTRIDIUM DIFFICILE (C. DIFF.) is a naturally occurring microbe in the human gut, one of many identified microbes that comprise the human microbiome. In a healthy body, C. diff. is unproblematic—it is a microbe that is relatively benign as part of the whole community. But when an individual takes a broad spectrum antibiotic medication, the microbial environment of the gut can change so as to wipe out many of the microbes that hold C. diff. in check; with their competition gone, C. diff. can bloom to the point of colonizing the gut. This leads to dysentery, and many individuals with C. diff. report having to go to the bathroom hourly in addition to needing to wear diapers to protect their clothing and furniture, a profound disruption akin to other disorders to the gut, bowels, and bladder.[1] As one might expect, C. diff. also leads to dehydration and malnourishment, and for many individuals who took antibiotics for a primary concern other than C. diff., this can be a life-threatening situation. The most thorough accounting of this patient population claims that about half a million Americans will have a C. diff. infection each year, and that about fifteen thousand of those will have a recurrent C. diff. infection, meaning that it fails to respond to first line treatment, which is to use another antibiotic.[2] These fifteen thousand patients are some of those seeking fecal microbial transplants (FMT), a treatment which proves to be about 90 percent effective.[3] Transfers can occur through two routes, the top or the bottom. In the case of a top procedure, a gavage tube is inserted nasally, and the transplant material is pumped past the stomach and into the intestine; in the case of a bottom procedure, an enema solution is prepared and inserted into the colon. Recently, experiments have been done with encapsulated FMT material that an individual swallows; the challenge is that, if a capsule dissolves due to stomach acid, the microbial infusion is lost in the stomach, never making it to the intestines where it would be therapeutic. In both top and bottom delivery of the FMT material, the patient is charged with holding the solution in their body for as long as possible, which can last minutes or hours depending on the constitution of the patient. The FMT solution is based on donor feces, often provided by a friend or family member of the patient, which has been tested for possible infectious microbes, blended with water and strained. The clinically preferred method of delivery is through the top, as it is generally assumed to be more effective,[4] but enema as a technique is easier and less objectionable to most patients, and is more popular particularly in cases of self-administration. The typical administration of the solution occurs daily, often for weeks at a time, although significant changes are reported by patients as soon as within twenty-four hours of treatment.

Given that many donations come from friends and family members and that the method of delivery is relatively easy, many individuals attempt self-administration. This is aided by websites like Power of Poop and several Facebook self-help groups, as well as many other websites and scientific papers that provide guidelines for testing donor feces and self-administration. Moreover, FMTs are not covered by many (if any) medical insurance plans in the United States, and physicians complain of lack of reimbursement for the procedure: they can fiddle with reimbursement codes, but cannot charge for the procedure as such, which has led to reports of patients paying as much as $10,000 for the procedure out of pocket. Since many patients are significantly beset by the C. diff. infection, they are willing to pay; or, if they are able and willing, treat themselves at home. During a period in the early 2010s in which the Food and Drug Administration (FDA) imposed an Investigative New Drug (IND) protocol restricting the use of FMTs to approved clinics, many patients conducted their own treatment, with or without clinical oversight, potentially leading to more risky procedures, harm to already sick individuals, and endangerment of the procedure's reputation and scientific validity.

In this chapter, I focus on a workshop held by the FDA and the National Institutes of Health (NIH) in May 2013 on the subject of FMT regarding their risks and clinical applicability.[5] By focusing on the ways that participants spoke in these meetings about the microbiome, individual bodies, and forms of treatment, I attend to how discursive registers are employed to produce bodily scales, from the smallest microbe to the body politic. Herein, I focus on how scale operates to conceptualize bodies, medical action, and the "colonial" project of FMT as a means to consider how scale serves medical governance. In so doing, the risks to the body politic associated with the human microbial colony become apparent, as do the problems with attempting to regulate these microbial colonies, and the people whom they inhabit. By focusing on this metaphorical "colony" and the registers through which medical professionals conceptualize bodies, disorders, and treatments—the "normal," the "regular," and the "standard"—some of the limits of contemporary medical governance can be elucidated, especially that individuals are much easier to control than microbial colonies are. In a context where microbial colonies are determinative of human health, but in which there is no definitive ability to control the colony or its effects, medical governance that has focused on the body and its containment in skin becomes thwarted and in need of reconceptualizing what a body is and how it is shaped. Regulating the colony within provides the ability to regulate individual bodies and society as a whole; what might at first appear to be a societal blip and rare occurrence in the debates about FMT opens up appreciation for how the microbial and excrement as medical substances have become subject to widespread concerns about purity and danger. To situate these debates, I turn back to the historical elaboration of the "medical police," a public health agency focused on the management of health risks, which never succeeded in the United States. Yet, the failure of the medical police as an institution points to the problems that the state faces in attempting to control the behaviors of individuals and the exposures they encounter in their everyday lives.

## What's at Stake in the FMT Debate?

The NIH-FDA workshop featured talks by scientists, clinicians, an entrepreneur, and regulatory officials from the FDA, all focused on the perceived risks and benefits of FMT. The NIH and FDA initiated the meetings due to a surge in popularity of FMT around 2011, used primarily as a treatment for C. diff. infections and based on the low risk and high success rate of FMT. At the time of the workshop in 2013, the FDA had recently imposed the need for clinicians to file an Investigative New Drug (IND) application for the use of FMT, effectively curtailing the ability of clinicians to use the treatment outside of large research hospitals with the staffing to prepare the hundreds-of-pages-long IND application. Of the many attendees, only one, Catherine Duff, was a prior recipient of FMT, and her testimony came at the end of the two-day workshop in an open question and answer period, not as a formal presentation:

> I'm one of those people who call and email you everyday. I've had eight episodes of recurrent C. diff and it's now antibiotic-resistant. I cannot find a doctor who will perform an FMT so my husband and I did it at home ourselves. Within 24 hours my symptoms were gone and I remained symptom and toxin-free until the next time I had to take antibiotics.
>
> At that time, one of my team of physicians agreed to perform an FMT without knowing what an IND was, that one was required, or that a [Current Procedural Terminology] code had been assigned. He did perform it in his surgical outpatient clinic and again within 24 hours, I had no symptoms. I remain symptom-free and toxin-free as of October of last year.
>
> People are desperate for this treatment. As doctors, clinicians, researchers, administrators, you know the stories of your patients, but you have not lived our lives. You have not felt our dwindling hope and our growing sense of despair. I now wonder each and every day if I will be able to have another one if needed, what I will do if it ceases to work, and what will I do if I encounter a different superbug.
>
> Currently physicians use many, many biologics. The risks are explained to and generally accepted by the patient. Speaking for the hundreds of thousands of people that cannot be here today, please go forward, be bold, be courageous, find a way to quickly, without several years of preclinical and clinical trials, allow qualified doctors to perform FMT with tested donors and signed consents without fear of regulatory consequences.
>
> If your spouse, child, parent, sibling, or best friend were dying

from antibiotic resistant C. diff, I imagine that all of you would want them to be able to try FMT and I imagine that most of you would agree to be the donor and to even perform the procedure yourself if necessary. People are dying everyday, today, right now.

I have a wonderful husband, three amazing daughters, and two small grandchildren, and I want to live. All of us just want a chance to live. Please, do something not only for me, but for all those around the country and everywhere who have no insurance, no financial resources, no computer with which to Google information, and no hope. Please do something quickly.

Duff lays out what is at stake in the workshop and the FDA's disallowance of clinicians to use FMT as a treatment through a shared sense of desperation: the FDA is afraid of the consequences of the treatment for individual patients and their physicians, who may face legal malpractice suits. Yet physicians are willing to perform FMTs because they recognize it as relatively safe and effective, and patients are willing to adopt the risks associated with FMTs because they are facing a humiliating, debilitating, and potentially life-threatening disorder. With the new IND paperwork requirements in place, the FDA effectively shut down access to FMTs for patients living anywhere but near major research hospitals. This resulted in many patients self-administering FMTs with the help of friends and relatives, a much riskier situation than seeking a medical professional. Along with Duff's moving testimony, these factors might be enough to dismantle the IND restrictions, but in this chapter I point to some of the scientific testimony that even further troubles the ability of the FDA and physicians to regulate individual behavior and treatment outcomes, all of which revolves around the constitution of the microbiome as risky, dirty, and dangerous, and invokes its potential disordering effects on American everyday life. Humans may be easy to govern, but the microbiome is much more unruly.

Given Duff's testimony, the results discussed by the clinicians and scientists at the workshop, and the risk of self-administered FMTs, the FDA eventually decided to "exercise enforcement discretion," effectively allowing clinicians to perform FMTs with only the informed consent of the patient at certain hospitals and clinics, thereby circumventing the

IND restrictions. Despite intense regulation and fear associated with medical malpractice and the discrediting of the science used to support FMTs as a procedure, the FDA decided to allow FMTs to proceed unimpeded by governmental regulation because of two factors: first, it had become challenging to govern patients and their access to medical techniques and knowledge, as made evident in Duff's and others self-administration of FMT; and, second, the human microbiome, which FMT relies on, fundamentally troubles medical governance in its unruliness. The modern U.S. state, which has never had a firm hold on the governance of medicine and its practice, is increasingly losing control due to the decentralization of medical practice through support networks, mail-order drugs, complementary and alternative medicine, and the dawning reality of the body's irreducibility; the microbial communities that make up a human's microbiome defy any easy attempt at control, either environmentally or chemically. The testimony of the clinicians and scientists at the NIH workshop point to this reality, although indirectly; throughout the proceedings, presenters offered images of microbial communities as unpredictable, unknowable, and difficult to manage for individual patients and medical staff. Rather than the transparent governance that grounds much of modern American biomedicine—which often occurs through providing access to specific treatments through physician approvals and medical insurance coverage—FMT and the human microbiome expose how governance fails to capture all communities, human and not, that make up the modern populations that comprise the body politic. We have entered an era of what Heather Paxson names "microbiopolitics,"[6] but without the apparatuses to predictably govern the forms of life that make up the microbial world we are a part of, either chemically or politically.

Through metaphor and everyday idioms, medical professionals talk about and conceptualize the body and its relation to FMT. This includes the metaphor of "colonization," which is used to construct the patient's body as a passive, transparent medium to receive an FMT treatment, the goal of the treatment being to render the patient "normal" as an individual body. The abnormal is regularized through a consideration of what "normal" looks like when brought to bear on the human digestive system. The human gut depends on "regularity" in a temporal frame, at the level of the microbial, physiological, clinical, and institutional, which is based in the long history of American interest in nutrition and regular bowel movements, echoing John Harvey Kellogg, Adelle Davis, and Benjamin Spock. The movement from "regular" to "standard" is principally informed by concerns about the market. Standardized products are sought to make human bodies "regular," working from the body's microbial constituents to the individual body. From the normal, to the regular, to the standard, patients, physicians, and researchers are scaling down, conceptualizing smaller levels of scale, their determinative effects on health, and how they might be acted on. They also scale up, focusing on the health of microbial communities to explain the health of individuals, and sometimes whole societies. "Normal," "regular," and "standard" are generally taken to be synonyms, but as demonstrated by the NIH-FDA proceedings, each has a valence shaped by ideas about the level of analysis that is being discussed by physicians and researchers. Moreover, "regularity" has a long history of associations with timing human eating and excretion. In tracking the shifts between these frames, the scale that is used to conceptualize the body and its iterations becomes apparent, as does the conceptual mechanisms through which shifts in scale are made when discussing microbes and their bodily interactions. In making these shifts, the body is constructed through medicine and science as existing in tension between, on the one side, a medically governed body as one of many similar bodies that are metonymic of the body politic, and on the other, the microbial body comprised of a population of unruly and unknown potentials that defy medical, scientific, and lay conceptions of discretely bounded human bodies.

FMT and gastroenterology offer a model of medicine as a colonial practice, as they often rely on metaphors about "community" and "colonization" to conceptualize the target and effects of microbial-based disease and their potential therapies. This language is at once metaphorical and based in the reality of medical practice: microbes are colonizing bodies with the goal of displacing the existing microbial community and replacing it with a new one. As a site of colonization, and comprising a native population, albeit of microbes, the human body is subject to medical governance, as is its microbiome. Humans, as long as they are compliant with the expectations of medical professionals and insurers, tend to be easily governed. But microbial communities prove much more difficult, as they are not only unpredictable in their reactions to treatment, but difficult even to document: there is no microbial census, and recent attempts to map the gut's genome cannot definitely describe which microbes are positive or negative for an individual's health.[7] In focusing on these communities, questions are raised about medical governance as it is applied to microbial bodies. By focusing on the microbial, the difficulties of modern medical governance are exposed, showing how the regulation of life on multiple scales—from the microbial to the individual body to the more-than-human community of society—becomes desirable and, ultimately, unattainable.

As it becomes difficult for medical professionals and the U.S. government to control the behaviors of individuals, particularly in the case of self-administering FMTs, as discussed throughout the NIH-FDA proceedings, recourse is made by clinicians, scientists, and bureaucrats involved in the NIH-FDA workshop to "standardization" provided by capitalist investment in manufacturing therapies that will produce governable subjects through medical intervention at the level of consumer products. This is apparent in the workshop by the interest in producing FMT kits that will produce "normal" microbial colonies in their recipients, and thereby render the individual body normal as well. As scholars of American medicine have shown, there is a strong trend in medicine toward the normalization of individual patients. This can be demonstrated by pharmaceuticals that shape affect, particularly antidepressants, but also treatments that shape everyday behaviors, like sleep, menstruation, and reproduction.[8] "Standardization" plays a vital role in the capitalization of consumer goods that are intended to maintain health and the normal functioning of the individual.[9] Similarly, presenters at the FMT workshop used "standardization" particularly in relation to the development of specific kinds of FMT kits to be bought by patient-consumers; they also used it to think through the contents of any particular microbial community and whether it was reflective of a "normal" human microbiome. In both cases, what was central to their conception of the microbiome was the individual human body of the patient and how a patient might be turned into a healthy individual through "colonization" with FMT. By conceptualizing the microbial as determinative of an individual's health, the participants in the NIH-FDA workshop were trafficking between the scale of the individual body and that of its microbial constituents. The right, possibly standardized, microbial community would produce a normal individual, or so proponents of FMT argued, and it might potentially scale up to the right body politic, a view similar to Kellogg's and Davis's early-twentieth-century euthenics. In these ways, FMT is haunted by the long history of racism related to medicine and microbes, and bodies and their substances, that have animated American medicine, which has structured the limits of the possible.

### From Abnormal to Regular: Stabilizing the Microbial Body through Temporal Patterning

In this section, I draw on speakers at the NIH-FDA workshop who each use the "normal" as a way to conceptualize the microbial colony inhabiting a human body, and how these colonies determine the normalcy (or lack thereof) of the individual body. With this basis of the normal, speakers then discuss the need to "regulate" the microbial colony, individual body, and institutional demands as a way to temporally situate the normal; through "regulation," the normal unifies bodies across scales, from the microbial to the individual to the institutional, echoing Kellogg and a century of American conceptions of self-regulation.

During the FDA proceedings, Lita Proctor, the director of the Human Microbiome Project, provided an example of how the normal comes to be used to conceptualize the microbial body, its internal changes, and their influences on the individual body. Foundational here is how the normal and the healthy become rendered as isomorphic, and how "healthy" becomes a mechanism to reduce the individual to the microbial.

> It's very hard to define healthy. So, the way that the [Human Microbiome Project] defined healthy was to actually consult a wide variety of specialists in each part of the body and talk to them about what would they consider a healthy or a normal condition of that body site. And so, a combination of inclusion and exclusion criteria were utilized to define healthy in this kind of super-healthy or carefully vetted cohort.[10]

During the question-and-answer session following her presentation, Proctor went on to explain: "I would have to say [the participants] were young and they were super healthy. So, yes, that's not necessarily the same thing as normal. Right? Right."[11] "Healthy" is taken as equal to "normal" when referring to the individual and one's microbial body; "super healthy," which she uses to refer to the participants in the Human Microbiome Project who had been carefully screened for microbe-impacting conditions or behaviors, is expressly set against the normal: the "super healthy" are not normal, but help to show what the expectations for medical research are, and who counts when it comes to developing knowledge about the human body.

Among the many presenters were a small number of animal microbiologists and veterinarians. Among veterinarians, FMT has a long-standing role in everyday practice, where it is referred to as "transfaunation."[12] To the extent that large mammals provide models of human biology, veterinary science provides a parallel set of evidence that is coming to be interpreted as relevant for addressing FMT among human populations. Linda Mansfield, a microbiologist from Michigan State University, provides a view of how many large animals are affected by transfaunation, leading to what she refers to as "a new normal" after illness and a period of treatment:

> If we look at the relationships between these microbial communities from different times we see that in pet one, on day one, these samples in these early samples before diarrhea clustered together, whereas during diarrhea and treatment they clustered differently. And then after resolution of the diarrhea they were in an entirely different group. And so, it's likely that there's a new normal associated with this [treatment].[13]

This "new normal" is both at the level of the microbial body, where a new colony has been established through the FMT procedure, and at the level of the individual and social body, in that the material conditions and social phenomenology of everyday life are shaped by the changes in microbial communities. As much as normalcy cuts across scale here, from the view of microbial science, the microbial body becomes an actor in this model, where the microbial colonies that exist within the individual body are conceptualized as materially shaping the body's capacities, particularly around eating, drinking, and excreting.

The effect of the microbial body and its relation to normalcy are also demonstrated through an anecdotal case presentation by University of Minnesota gastroenterologist Alex Khoruts, a leader in the field of experimental FMT who has been key in the technique's resurgence since the early 2000s. His NIH-FDA presentation focused primarily on the efficacy of the treatment, but he highlighted exceptional cases where FMT was less than wholly effective, as in the following:

> In this third patient here, it was kind of interesting, around day 28 . . . there is some expansion of proteobacteria and then there is a bigger expansion, and what happened here is a bladder infection, and actually the antibiotic was initiated a little bit after this expansion was noted. . . . This patient did not normalize within the three months that we studied her afterwards, after that episode of getting bacterium and having her [urinary tract infection].[14]

As Khoruts points out, the microbial body is unpredictable in its effects, and although FMT proves particularly efficacious when used to treat C. diff., it is unclear what side effects it may have—and what other conditions it might interfere with the treatment of, as the microbial communities on and in the human body interact in unpredictable ways. In the case of this patient, who is diagnosed with a urinary tract infection and treated for it with antibiotics, the expectations of her progression related to the FMT treatment are disrupted by the introduction of antibiotics that affect the microbial communities of her body. As a result, she does "not normalize" as might be expected of another FMT recipient. Here, the microbial body and the individual body are brought together through the idiom of the normal, a scalar operation that runs parallel to the use of ideas about "regulation," particularly as it relates to the governable body politic.

Through the language of the speakers at the FDA hearing, "regulation" is posited to exist at the level of cells, organs, and on the other end of the scale, institutions like the FDA and human-subject review boards in hospitals. Moving between these levels of scale allow bodies to be thought of both at the molecular level and at the level of the body politic, as "regulation" collapses conceptions of agentive power as it relates to the body and one's ability to control bodies and their operations through deliberate governance. At the level of the molecular body, consider the discussion by Yasmine Belkaid, chief of the Mucosal Infection Section of the NIH, of "regulatory T cells" in the human gut:

> If you actually take some regulatory T cells that reside in the gut and if you actually look at the specificity of these T regs, [a] certain fraction of these cells [are] actually specific for commensal antigens. So, this is a very important feature of the regulatory pathway of the GI tract.[15]

Belkaid's description and use of "regulation" are molecular in their conception; she suggests that the body is shaped by the functions of physiological features like cells, hormones, and antibodies. Compare this to the conception of regulation that David Rubin, professor of medicine at the University of Chicago, presents of regulation in the gut as a crisis of broader social transformations and their impacts on the body, particularly the "hygiene hypothesis":

> The hygiene hypothesis postulates that the environment has become too clean, that our guts are designed to interact with our environment or to be infected or coexist with parasites in some ways and that when we're younger, we have a developmental phase in our immune system that no longer is exposed to the right things to train it to respond properly, and when we become young adults and we do get exposed to something, there's this turned-on immune response in the gut that loses its ability to regulate, and that's what we call [irritable bowel disorder].[16]

Rubin scales down, moving between the social management of dirt and disease to the functioning of specific bodies that have been impacted by this change in the ecology that humans are a part of; he also scales up, blaming large-scale epidemiological concerns on the changes humans have collectively made to their microbial environments. "Regulation" moves from the macro to the micro, implicating the macro for shaping the micro, but these macro-level efforts are shaped by the presence of the molecular and microbial: the push toward hygiene is founded in a conception of human life as being shaped by the existence of forces too small for the eye to see, and too small to act on except through similarly micro-focused mechanisms.

This move toward the regulation of society through broad governmental public-health efforts regarding hygiene points to the need to shape the institutional decision-making that may result in effects like those ascribed to the overuse of antibiotics and antibacterial soap, the foundation of the hygiene hypothesis and its attempt to explain the increase of disease as a result of lack of exposures to nature. As is made clear by Lee Jones, the CEO of Rebiotix, a microbiota-focused start-up, the need to regulate behaviors of individuals and institutions by other institutions is in the service of controlling the outcomes of the use of experimental procedures like FMT. For Jones, as an entrepreneur invested in the development of a "standardized" kit to provide a reproducible and marketable product, the danger in not having regulation is something that may have negative effects both for individual bodies and capitalist efforts.

> Regulations and quality standards have a very important role to play. They do two major things for all of us, they protect the patient, and because they do that, they protect the industry. This [patient-conducted FMT] is one of those things that if it runs amok and has a disaster, it's going to be hard to recover from because people will lose faith that this is something that could be helpful.[17]

Jones's invocation of "quality standards" is an appeal for standardization, the adoption of particular ways of producing products and experimenting with them. These quality standards are shaped by institutional regulations but are also meant to lead to particular kinds of molecular and microbial regulation. The danger that Jones anticipates is less about the individual patient and more about the corporate interests that he speaks on behalf of: the damage to a patient from an unsuccessful or harmful FMT is less important to him than what effect the mediatization of this event will have on the ability to pursue FMT as a viable, marketable treatment for C. diff. and related complaints. The need, Jones argues, is to embrace standardization through regulation, thereby preserving the ability for biomedicine to act on the body at its many conceptual scales, from the tiny microbe, to the multitudinous microbial colony, to the body in its social environment. Regulation is based on the acceptance of the body as landscape, the need to govern what a body is exposed to and how a body is changed in relation to these exposures.

## From Regular to Standard: Making the Body Normal through Capitalist Standardization

The movement from the regular to the standard is one that requires a conception of the institutionally governed body politic as having profound effects on the behaviors of individuals, both at the level of their social interactions and at the level of their microbial and molecular bodies. Standardization relies on the possibility of regulation, whether on the level of biological products like FMT treatments or on that of individuals, and is embedded in the processes of institutions and their determinative powers. However, the only direct control that can be exerted on a microbial community is through other microbial communities and molecular compounds, and these are inexact in their effects, which lays the basis for the unruliness of microbial communities. At its most efficacious, standardization works across scales, normalizing a microbial community, the body it inhabits, and the medical institutions that make these effects possible. Barry Eisenstein, senior vice president of scientific affairs at Cubist Pharmaceuticals, made this clear when he asked during the NIH-FDA workshop: "But how are you going to regulate the individual at home who calls one of the gastroenterologists and tries to get some advice? I don't understand how that works?"[18] This question, directed at representatives of the NIH and FDA, is a question about regulating both the behavior of patients and that of physicians and other medical professionals in a position to provide potential patients with FMT as a medical treatment. This depends, in turn, on the existence of a standard to which FMT treatments, in their composition, can be held; a nonstandardized treatment, as in the use of a family member or friend as a donor, even in the hands of a physician, may lead to unwelcome outcomes, or so the fears expressed by speakers at the NIH-FDA workshop index. What follows is the implication that pharmaceutical companies might provide a means to make the lives of both medical professionals and patients easier by providing a standardized mechanism to produce a desired outcome. This depends on making FMT a viable treatment, as well as making human fecal material something that can be considered a product that can be regulated and standardized, an effort that depends on the FDA and its classification of biological materials suitable for therapeutic use.

The central standardization problem for the FDA is what FMT, and human feces in particular, counts as: is feces used in the context of an FMT a drug or a biological product? To count as a biological product, the biological substance need only be modified before its introduction into another body, which is a problem of standardizing the microbial to normalize the individual body. As Jay Slater, the director of the Division of Bacterial, Parasitic, and Allergenic Products at the FDA explains, reading from official documentation, biological products include

> "a virus, therapeutic serum, toxin, antitoxin, vaccine, blood, blood component or derivative, allergenic product, protein, or analogous product"—I know you were all waiting to see where fecal material fit in—"or analogous product, applicable to the prevention, treatment, or cure of a disease or condition in human beings."[19]

What makes fecal material even more problematic is that it changes from day to day, from sample to sample, which makes it different from biologics like blood. One donation can vary significantly from another, and even from the same person, based on changes in diet and environmental exposures; the result is that there is routine variation within the microbiota in feces. Moreover, unlike a blood transfusion that, with appropriate screening, is accepted as having no contagious influence between donor and recipient, the purpose of FMT is to make the gut of the recipient more like, if not identical to, that of the donor, a process that takes only days. Khoruts explains: "Usually three days [after the procedure] is when we have the first bowel movement that we can count on collecting. It looks virtually identical to that of the donor. And that persists."[20] Because of these two forces—that donor microbial communities vary over time and that they have a profound mimetic influence on the recipient—the goal expressed by many of the scientists, and made explicit by one industry representative, was to make a "standard" kit of microbiota to establish "normal" gut health based on a select group of proven microbial colonizers.

As Eisenstein from Cubist Pharmaceuticals makes clear, there are obvious rationales for the move toward an industrially manufactured, "standardized" FMT product. Much like Jones above, Eisenstein accepts that the push toward industrially manufacturing FMT products is both a safety concern and a necessary basis for the commercialization of the procedure and related products:

> There seems to be a continuum from the non-physician homebrew to the doc's office that is making use of non-standardized material to the more standardized medical centers, . . . to the industrial commercialization product, to, then later, an understanding of how we would use an artificial mixture of very well defined individual components that could be put together that for all time would then be active pharmaceutical product that would then be studied. And it seems that going from one end of the continuum to another, you're getting increasing characterization, increasing standardization, and increasing opportunity to better study and understand potency and efficacy and safety and also increasing opportunities to commercialize.[21]

Similarly, Colleen Kelly, assistant professor of medicine at Brown University, echoes the likelihood that it will be the pharmaceutical industry, not hospital-based research centers, that will lead the way toward standardization:

> I think what we're all going towards is some kind of a standardized product that's easy and safe and studies can be duplicated and results are more consistent, and I think that that's probably going to happen through industry rather than magic fairies coming down and giving us money to do it.[22]

This push toward commercialized, mass-produced FMT products is simultaneously a push toward a normative conception of the human body and the relative ease with which one body can be substituted for another through the mediation of a standardized product. It is precisely through the language of standardization that capitalist interests are able to control the body: medicine often traffics in conceptions of the normal that refer primarily to the individual body and its material status, but standardization depends on a conception of the normal and the means to produce it through industrial processes and products, working from the microbial or molecular up to the individual body. Standardization depends on static, reproducible outcomes that are founded in the normal but are made possible through manufacture and assumptions about bodily transparency and plasticity.

This promise of standardization informs capitalist technoscience. As Jones explains, Rebiotix is "solving the problems of FMT by providing and developing a commercialized, standardized, ready-to-use product." Thus, rather than rely on donor networks, which often depend on kinship ties, Jones and the scientists at Rebiotix are attempting to produce a universal transplant based on the donations of five individuals. There are two problems, however. First, an audience member suggests that "what we consider as normal may not be normal hosts; normal or supposedly healthy people may not truly be healthy. They may actually become diseased very soon."[23] That is, due to the complexity of the microbiota, what may look normal could be obscuring pending disorders, which may eventually become evident both in the donor and the recipient. Second is the very important point that the power of the microbiota is not based on one, three, or ten specific microbes, but rather the synergistic powers of the entire microbial "community." The goal, as Vincent Young from the University of Michigan claims, is "to restore a good community and replace a bad community."[24] The cure that microbial transfusions offer is not conversion based on lone microbial missionaries, but rather full-scale colonization, leading to the normalization of the individual body.

## Diffuse Threats Call for Direct Policing

The NIH-FDA workshop was responding to the microbiopolitical context that FMTs were being explored in by FMT seekers and health-care providers. With the growing awareness of the human microbiome and the role of microbes in human life more generally, what was once a biopolitical project that focused on whole, molar bodies became focused, instead, on the microbial actors that were moving between bodies. Attention to these microscopic vectors was facilitated through new laboratory technologies that allowed for their visualization, containment, and DNA sequencing. As scientific objects, even though knowledge about microbes was over a century old,[25] their powers had to be accounted for; this animated concerns about how microbes might transmit chronic illnesses, like type 2 diabetes and hepatitis, even though many panelists in the workshop understood that to not be possible, given the current state of microbial science. But this was possible because, in the newly increased knowability of microbes, these vectors also became increasingly unknown: What else could their powers be? And how could those powers be regulated? In seeking to address these concerns, the NIH and FDA were forced to confront their mandates to protect public health as well as the health of individuals, which brought to the surface how disgust as a bureaucratic affect has long animated American institutions charged with protecting the health of its people.

Before the FDA, there were other medical institutions that sought to control populations through their exposures to risky substances. One of these institutions, which never succeeded in the United States, was that of the "medical police." Developed by Johann Peter Frank in his *A System of Complete Medical Police,*[26] the medical policeman—and I use the gendered term here to flag the historicity of the term as defined and promulgated by Frank—was specifically intended to enforce emerging standards of civilization, particularly in the booming urban centers of industrializing Germany and Austria in the eighteenth and nineteenth centuries, as part of the Cameralist interest in *Polizei.*[27] Rather than focus on legal statutes per se, the medical police were intended to enforce scientific and medical best practices later codified as hygienic, some of which would become foundational in determining what forms legal statutes should take, particularly related to the care of waste. Frank's concept of the medical police ultimately failed on two fronts: first, it failed to become a common aspect of governance throughout the North Atlantic, and especially the United States; second, the *Polizei* became the legally focused, violence-enabled police, rather than the hygienically focused public-health workers or bureaucrats, as in the FDA.[28] *Polizei,* eventually rendered *policy,* comes to stand for the law, associated most strongly with the emergent institutions of modernity in the North Atlantic, to which nature was portrayed as oppositional and in need of taming not through the law, but through medicine and science, as through the FDA. Attention to the failures of the medical police as a concept and set of practices brings into relief the role of the human body and its care in contemporary U.S. law, policy, and public opinion, particularly as informed by emerging ideas of corporeality, disease, and individuality in the context of American modernity, founded in ideas about the body and disease, a charge that the FDA would assume in the control of substances used as medicines and the care for the American body politic through regulation.

As formulated by Frank in the late eighteenth century, the medical police were concerned with the promulgation of health, which led them to environmental interventions like making sure that people tended to animal and human waste, the draining of swamps, and other miasmatic threats, as well as the monitoring of agricultural production and the storage of foodstuffs. The Austro-German institution of medical police succeeded Swedish efforts to promote vitality and fertility and paralleled other paternalistic efforts to promote health and life throughout western and central Europe, as well as Great Britain, all of which were biopolitical efforts.[29] But in the United States, there were no medical police, despite the medical police's integral function in the development of an industrial working class and its livelihood in Europe. Instead, in the United States throughout the late eighteenth and nineteenth century, "boards of health" and similarly titled institutions were convened only in response to epidemic disease and other explicit, widespread threats, which often came from Europe by ship, at which point citizens and civil servants adopted the mandate to clean cities, quarantine the sick, and otherwise maintain a sanitary society.[30] As Charles Rosenberg describes in the context of cholera outbreaks in the United States, after the proximate threat had passed, these civic-governmental structures and their activities decayed, leading to a lapse in the individual and environmental oversight needed to avoid another epidemic, which would, inevitably, help ensure another wave of epidemic disease, including yellow fever in the 1790s and waves of cholera throughout the 1800s.

Only by the end of the nineteenth century would these organizational forms become durable, leading to the eventual development of "public health" as a societal necessity and the governance of public health through institutions like the FDA and Centers for Disease Control (CDC).[31] But public health was unpoliced, falling into a zone of indeterminacy in which it is unclear which authority has the power to enforce laws and what enforcement entails. By "unpoliced," I mean to flag the ways that particular kinds of behaviors and social concerns escape the notice of police and may also be uncodified by local legal statutes, like the discreet use of FMT by wily treatment seekers. For example, if a person actually did a home FMT, what law would they be breaking? A willing health-care provider who aided in the delivery of FMT might be sued for malpractice if something went awry, or might have their insurance billing refused, but they too are not breaking a law in the strict sense, even with the FDA's regulations in place. Inasmuch as the FDA can seek to exert control, it relies on a bureaucratic form of power that has few teeth. Instead, FMT might be imagined as being "unpoliced." Using "unpoliced" in this context is a way to convey that a set of actions elide easy legal capture and legal enforcement due to their absence as directly codified in law. This is not to suggest that these practices evade the law altogether, since there are multiple ways that actions can be construed to fit into existing laws; but, if they are to be captured in the law, additional labor needs to be done to make them subject to police intervention through the powers of the FDA and related agencies.

In considering why the medical police never translated to the U.S. context, the contradictions of health and the law in the United States come into stark relief: health and disease are construed as intensely individual. Not-quite-criminal choices made by sick individuals that affect the social fabric in harmful ways—particularly members of the same family and local environment—are difficult to attribute to a culpable individual. One counterexample might be the knowing exposure of an individual to a life-threatening, communicable disease, such as HIV, where this action is construed as a form of murder or assault.[32] But in the United States, limiting the movement and actions of individuals through an institution like medical police is taken as an undue burden on the personal liberty of individuals; instead, ancillary institutions like departments of public health tend to this aporia in legal structure, but through means that may or may not be explicitly based in codified law, except in cases where direct harm can be proven and the threat to health is demonstrable and evident, which is what the NIH-FDA workshop sought to accomplish. Without strict codification and penalties, health-threatening behaviors are difficult to deter. In much the same way that other forms of criminality have been historically conceived, the noncrimes associated with disease transmission, while construed as congenital in the eighteenth and nineteenth centuries (as associated with kinds of people based on race, ethnicity, disability, and class), are now conceived of as due to economic disenfranchisement, but in all cases associated with dirt and disorder in ways that uphold the exclusion of individuals and communities. This is true at the institutional level, and as discussed in chapter 6, at the personal level.

Frank is representative of proponents of scientific medicine in his generation and lays out the ways that disease is influenced by environmental conditions that could be easily curtailed by deliberate, modernist efforts at being more civilized:

> Who does not know the devastating scourge of hospital fever, hospital infection, and typhoid epidemics which have their origin here! These very volatile animal products escape from the sick organism by way of breath, saliva, sweat, urine and excrement, or rather all the excretions are mixed with miasmas; they have the most devastating effect on the live organism and produce terrible general epidemics. Miasmas develop from rotting animal and vegetable substances. Unburied or not deeply enough buried human and animal bodies, animal waste in slaughterhouses, butchers' stalls, tanneries, soap works, in factories producing gut strings, etc., latrines, manure pools, peat bogs, flax and hemp roasting, etc., are the sources of such poisonous vapors. . . . The deleterious miasmas were received by the atmosphere and spread their nefarious effect over mankind.[33]

Frank, like many of his contemporaries, and many natural philosophers and early modern physicians, supported the miasmatic theory of disease transmission, which echoed ideas about sympathetic magic, miasmas making disease because of the qualities of the air and its intake by unsuspecting breathers. In an era before the identification of bacteria and viruses, miasmatic theory relied on the understanding of "bad air" leading to disease. Miasmas were natural, if dangerous, products of the world, intensified by dense human habitation, where masses of human-produced waste would intermingle and generate bad air. These miasmas could also be naturally occurring, in swamps and other conducive environments; in earlier times, individuals were warned away from travel through particular areas due to the local existence of such miasmatic formations. Moreover, a miasma might travel, spreading disease in its circulation through the atmosphere. The emerging urban centers of Europe and the United States meant that the careless management of human-produced waste (trash, offal, shit, corpses) both could be generated more easily through density of population and would potentially be more insidious and lethal due to easier methods of transmission and infection. This affected people living in close proximity to these miasmas, and also those living in close quarters with poor ventilation, which led, as Frank notes, to miasmatic formations in their own right. Those particularly prone to the careless management of waste that produces miasmas were generally construed to be the illiterate and poor working classes, who failed to understand the basic science of disease transmission. The medical police were intended to intervene into this ignorance, enforcing scientific and social standards of waste removal and care, thereby upholding the edifice of civilization. This legacy informs the practice of the FDA, CDC, and NIH as they seek to protect the public from emergent dangers.

The medical police and early public-health-focused bureaucrats were integral in producing the urban geographies of the emerging industrial landscapes in western and central Europe, both in city centers and in the rural areas that serviced these urban centers in the production of food and laborers. Critical in Frank's conception of developing a healthy landscape was removing and isolating waste in centralized spaces, and in so doing, the removing of every trace of waste in the city itself. This upheld the idealized view of the city as the center of civilized society, despite its likely exposure to the many miasmatic threats spawned by close habitation. This purification of space was not to simply police what belongs where, but to police the movement of bodies and waste through space and to tie the existence of waste to the behaviors of individuals:

At a certain distance from all human dwellings and public roads, and if possible at a place from which the wind may not so easily blow into town, every town must maintain several reservoirs for the rubbish brought there from the town. In Paris, two kinds of receptacles are filled, one with real excrement, the other with other objects easily subject to rotting, dead animals, entrails, blood, rotten plants, etc.

The drivers conveying such materials must be strictly instructed not to empty any of these on the way into rivers, depressions, or onto fields; that they load the rubbish without delay at night into well closed barrels, and drive off before daybreak, after having previously swept clean the place where the loading took place; that under no pretext do they stop on the way and dirty the streets, etc.[34]

Whereas miasmas were diffuse, and sometimes mysterious in their origins and effects, Frank worked to situate them in space and particular human behaviors, providing medical police with specific targets for their powers. Like other forms of criminality, specific spatiotemporally situated behaviors became isomorphic with the intents of individuals: for Frank, those behaviors that act as a direct threat to society are those most in need of policing through the medical police. It is precisely in the intersection between individual self-determination and threats to a greater society where the medical police are meant to operate—they are not intended to police abstract or indirect threats—but it is in this intersection that their powers are most threatened, and it would be at these intersections that later bureaucracies like the FDA sought to aim their powers.

Frank argues that, while egocentric interest in self-determination is proposed as the key by which the rational practice of medical police could successfully shape all of society, it is also the barrier that must be overcome to do so.

> I compared with admiration our times with those olden times, when the great lawgiver dealt with the lowliest detail to such an extent that he even ordered that every Israelite in camp should have his little shovel with him, with which to cover carefully his excrement with soil. Nowadays much more important proposals on medical matters immediately evince sayings such as: "Well, yes, how can this be done?" "This is too petty for the police to bother about it! . . . ." "That way everybody would have his hands bound, etc." However, basically, we are simply too lazy to do good, and we value too highly every step that is required of us for the sake of the public weal.[35]

This problem of self-determination, however central it is to the very structure of criminality and the law, and Frank would argue, in need of policing, is the basis for the nonacceptance of medical police as a concept and set of practices in the United States, a tension that is recurrent in public health and the regulation of medical treatment, especially vaccination and complementary and alternative medicines. As an example, in 1793, epidemic yellow fever in Philadelphia would put these assumptions about self-determination and health to the test. In lieu of medical police, "Guardians" came to the aid of the sick and poor, a class of young men with political aspirations who were tasked with helping to secure the city against threats to civic life.[36] Generally, the job of a Guardian was modest, albeit undesirable and accepted as a step toward greater public service and power in a lifelong political career. Those who served as Guardians were likely not wholly different from the medical police in disposition, but when epidemic yellow fever struck, as J. H. Powell recounts in his history of yellow fever, many of them abandoned their posts for fear of becoming sick. The "public weal" suffered for lack of policing, which may be the moral failing of individual Guardians, but in the context of the early United States, similar moral failings were apparent everywhere, from authorities leaving their posts, to port authorities accepting plague-ridden shipments, to the poor, disease-ridden urban citizens, all of whom were believed culpable in the spread of yellow fever and the deaths that ensued. When epidemic disease would strike again in the form of cholera throughout the U.S. Eastern Seaboard, as Charles Rosenberg has provided ample histories of, boards of health would arise based on the interests of individual citizens to preserve the "public weal," but this would serve as an extra-governmental institution invested in public health, property values, and personal rights, with the upper classes intervening on the behaviors and lifestyles of the urban poor and sick. Cholera and yellow fever were both diffuse threats, not unlike the miasmatic causes of disease Frank identified elsewhere, but under the mandates of the emerging boards of health throughout the nineteenth century, the interventions taken on the part of the those boards were directed at individuals perceived as sick or criminal as well as at the dirtiness of industrial, urban civilization. The individual became the site of intervention, both to protect the public weal and to protect themselves. In some cases, this meant direct intervention through policing and public health officials, but it could also rely on inculcating conceptions of the self and environment that uphold norms in diffuse and indirect ways. The legacies of these efforts and these governmental sentiments exist in the CDC, FDA, and NIH, all of which seek to regulate what we are exposed to and how those exposures happen, including whether those exposures might be considered medicinal in their purpose.

The duties of the medical police as outlined by Frank have been adopted piecemeal by other U.S. institutions, with some responsibilities like the monitoring for the care of others falling under the auspices of "departments of social welfare," others like the monitoring of food safety being associated with the FDA and U.S. Department of Agriculture, and the monitoring of disease being the responsibility of the CDC and local departments of public health. Such a dispersal of responsibilities and powers allows some actions like the use of FMT by desperate people to slip through the law, despite what might be taken as threats to individual well-being and public health. Because we have always been engaged in a form of unknowing microbiopolitics, it may seem that bodies, both human and nonhuman, have been able to be regulated through medical governance, as we substitute the molar, human body for all of its constituents. But, as microbiopolitics has a more nuanced view of these tiny actors, it becomes apparent that microbial life has always exceeded our abilities to control it. At best, we can regulate our exposures to it. But this is a burden we adopt as individuals—and an opportunity we might pursue through experimental procedures and novel dieting practices that recompose our bodies as landscapes that we tend to as knowing stewards of the colony within and its environmental embeddedness.

## Become Your Own Medical Police

With the rise of attention to multispecies relationships and their effects on human health, it is increasingly necessary to have models to conceptualize the many determinants of human health, including the microbial and molecular, and how they are framed by and shaped through everyday life and expert knowledge production. As made evident by FMT, patients and physicians, scientists and corporate leaders, are reckoning with the reality of human health in a multispecies world, particularly in relation to microbial communities that fundamentally shape the experience of individuals and ideas about normalcy. This means a redefinition of the human body and how it is composed, which includes the environments that shape individual bodies, from the microbial communities humans interact with, to epigenetic determinants of health and disease, to the industrially produced diets and pharmaceuticals that shape the body in particular ways, to the symbolic and political mechanisms through which these chemical and microbial realities are apprehended. As Amber Benezra and Jamie Lorimer have argued, albeit in different contexts and focused on different nonhuman actors, human health is increasingly being conceptualized as more-than-human and dependent on interactions between microbes, parasites, symbionts, and others.[37] Awareness of these connections broadens the terrain that is conceptualized as the foundation for individual and societal health, making care for nonhuman others essential to promote human well-being, thereby necessitating forms of stewardship that move beyond the human in the strict sense and toward the human as a feature in a multispecies landscape.

Public health's history is deeply imbricated in ideas about the excremental and the need to clean up bodies and spaces, which continues in FDA regulations regarding the use of biologics in medicine. Over that history, particular bodies and spaces have been constructed as necessarily threats to the social order and have been targeted for overt forms of policing and control. Just as importantly, diffuse ideas about disease and dirt have led to forms of self-regulation that ensure that individuals are acting in ways that uphold societal norms: certain foods are suspect or particular medical practices are discredited or cast as dangerous. In these cases, the symbolic valences of dirt allow practices and goods to be unpoliced—they fall into the legal zone of indeterminacy where individuals are left to police themselves. But because of the variability of situations that an individual might face, that individual is charged with making decisions based in emergent conditions and individual sensibilities, which are framed by disgust; this can lead to confrontations with disgust that limit the choices people make, precisely based in ideas about the preservation of order and the management of dirt, especially in relation to one's body. Those individualized choices, however, discretely reflect and enact widespread attitudes about dirt and disease that echo embedded, historically produced sentiments.

How scale operates in the conceptualization of the human body and its microbial determinants of health exposes what is at stake in governing FMT and the need for the government to exert control on bodies through legitimate medical procedures. By focusing on how scientists, physicians, entrepreneurs, and patients use idioms of the normal, the regular, and the standard in conceptualizing individual bodies and the microbial colonies that inhabit these bodies, as well as the ways they can be used to modify other microbial communities, it becomes evident how these interlocking concepts apply to the individual body, the microbial communities that individuals host, and the industrial and medical processes that ensure particular kinds of "normal" bodies are produced. By regulating microbial communities, bodily processes, social interactions, and institutional practices, normative spatiotemporal expectations might be achieved in individuals and society at large, but the production of normal bodies depends on standardizing medical practices and microbial communities, which in turn depends on rendering the human body as a site of colonization, at least at the level of the microbial. From this perspective, by standardizing the microbial (the human body at one of its smallest scales), a normal, individual body can be achieved, but this depends on isolating it as a vessel for colonization. Purifying the body in this way has depended on a history of environmental management that purifies the spaces that bodies exist within, taming them of their dirt, both real and symbolic.[38] This is accomplished through direct and indirect forms of regulation.

As Khoruts testifies, through microbial colonization, FMT makes individuals more like each other. Rather than making individuals more like their kin or close friends who might be donors, the push the FDA and microbiota start-ups embrace is for "standard," "normal" donors who provide "good" communities to replace the "bad" ones. There is significant commercial interest in developing "standard" FMT kits, which moves beyond their use solely in the case of C. diff. The Rebiotix website suggests the next targets are ulcerative colitis and metabolic syndrome,[39] and there have also been claims that the microbiota may be to blame for autism, as well as type 2 diabetes, which I return to in chapter 6. In an era of blockbuster drugs that routinely make $1 billion annually, fifteen thousand C. diff. patients each year is not enough to support a burgeoning industry, but if one adds the many other possibilities that FMT might treat, the horizon expands significantly. Just like many other treatments, the aim is to standardize the individual to normative ideals produced in a laboratory and concretized through cultural expectations. In this way, the microbial becomes fundamental to the biology of everyday life, serving as a means to create bodies that act and react in reliable ways through the regular ingestion of particular kinds of substances that produce predictable effects, much like pharmaceuticals are intended to do (when side effects are minimized or nonexistent).

The problem, however, is that a "good" microbial colony varies over time—there is no standard "good" community, but only good interactive potential, based on what people eat, the diseases they are exposed to, and the broader ecological milieu an individual is composed through. This is the root of the problem for medical governance: unlike so many pharmaceutical treatments that aim to make an individual fit the demands of modern U.S. society and are largely predictable in their positive and negative effects, successful FMT depends on the establishment of a community of microbes that changes over time, is flexibly responsive to environmental changes, and has synergistic properties that exceed biomedical reductionism. As such, the colony within defies governmental logics of normalization; by extension, governance that takes as its goal the production and maintenance of normal bodies through FMT is fundamentally thwarted, as there is no norm to aspire to, but only abstract potentiality embodied in a multitudinous community of microbes. Although FMT kits might produce a "standard" biomedical subject, even this new "standard" is a moving target. The question that remains is whether this marks one possible end of biomedical forms of control, or an opening into new regimes of regulation, to the extent that our microbiotic communities will tolerate governance of any sort, which FMT seekers will not, as I explore in chapter 6. Yet, disgust provides a diffuse way to ensure that microbial medicine will be rejected as medicine, thereby providing a means to police bodies and the medicines they employ without needing to directly intervene on individual decision-making processes. In this way, the medical police live on, but only through our inculcated senses of hygiene, disgust, and the dangers we viscerally apprehend as threats to our bodily integrity. But desperation can provoke the need to reconceptualize the terrain of possibilities, thereby recomposing the body and its relation to the microbial.

# Threshold 3
## DESPERATION ON THE CUSP OF DISGUST

IN MAY 2021, Jane Sullivan was interviewed by Lindsey Parsons of the *Perfect Stool* podcast.[1] Parsons is a certified health coach who specializes in the gut, through her High Desert Health business, and hosts the podcast, which features scientists, health-care providers, and individuals who share their health journeys and which often includes discussions of the use of fecal microbial transplants (FMT). In many cases, their use of FMT is clandestine and something that they embark on with limited or no clinical support. Instead, they have reached a point in their health journey where desperation motivates them to, as Parsons says, "take the plunge." Many of Parsons's conversations are with practiced storytellers who have told the tale of their experimentation with FMT with some regularity, a function of having to tell friends, family, and health-care providers about the transformations in their health. But Sullivan is a particularly charismatic guest, a well-practiced storyteller with an unconventional narrative about mental health and her being healed through the use of her partner's "unicorn" feces. Sullivan's case is also exceptional in that she successfully uses FMT to treat her bipolar disorder, which is not a condition that would normally be considered for treatment through microbial medicine. Sullivan offers an example of both what is possible with FMT and also why the future of microbial medicine is an impossible one. This impossibility is evident in Parsons's and Sullivan's discussions of their experiences of disgust, which grow out of the settler-colonial contexts they come from, Parsons from the American Southwest and Sullivan from Australia's outback. Both women are responding to excrement-in-the-present and the regimes of bodily disgust that are present in their social worlds; but both are also responding to human excrement and its settler-colonial histories.

FMT has been experimented with by clinicians and would-be patients alike for any numbers of conditions, including irritable bowel syndrome, Crohn's, celiac, and more controversially, autism and Alzheimer's. The risks are accepted as minimal, especially if a person can overcome the "ick factor" and can locate a safe and viable donor. The successes have been few and marginal for conditions beyond the strictly gastrointestinal, at least from the perspective of biomedical experts. Part of this is based in the accepted impossibility of being able to cure autism and complex medical problems that even traditional biomedicine cannot; yet, proponents suggest that a mitigation of symptoms might be possible. The growing evidence that the gut affects the brain, leading to careful diets, supports a form of self-regulation as stewardship that many families can accept and does not require FMT. When successes occur—and Sullivan is seemingly an unqualified success—this will always be the basis for discrediting the microbial: she is a specific case, a bundle of history, physiology, and microbiota that is one of a kind, even if she might share some of those elements with her kin. Moreover, her partner Alex and his microbiome are unique too, their powers of healing isolated to him alone, and to the interactions produced through his body's excreta and the bodies it colonizes through FMT. He is not an "ideal" or "super" donor in any conventional sense, but a complementary one that supplies Sullivan with what her body needs.

Sullivan's narrative is long, complicated, and graphic. She is the victim of sexual abuse early in her life and has experience of long bouts of violent mania and life-stunting depression. But her case is compelling because, for all of these complications, FMT works. Donations from Alex also work for her sisters, who have also been diagnosed with bipolar, and for her mother. But whether Alex's colonial infusions work because of or despite the complexities of Sullivan and her siblings' histories is unknowable, and because of the ongoing flux of symptoms, diet, and environmental influences, the knowability of what precisely is working and how will always remain elusive.

This is how Sullivan tells her early history:

> Growing up, I had quite a lot of adverse childhood experiences, you
> know, I had a very stressful childhood, my mother was physically and
> mentally ill, and that really affected her parenting ability. And that

caused significant trauma in my childhood, and then a lot of bullying. So it wasn't a happy childhood. But I was functional up until my mid-teens when I was, unfortunately, groomed and molested by my uncle. This trauma put me into a health spiral very shortly afterwards, and I developed chronic tonsillitis and then ended up taking multiple courses of antibiotics over a two-year period. . . . Shortly after the abuse is when I fell apart and became basically non-functional. The trauma, for sure, was the trigger for serious mental illness. But knowing what I know about the gut microbiome and then the success later with the FMT resolving my symptoms, I really think that the trauma probably was the stress that affected my immune system and made me ill, and then the multiple courses of antibiotics must have just knocked out my gut microbiome into a state of dysbiosis and knocked out some keystone species that were really important for mental health.

Sullivan accepts some prior psychiatric sensitivity, a predisposition to mental illness, which she shares with the women in her family. Her molestation by her uncle tipped her toward depression, but it is the chronic tonsillitis and the courses of antibiotics that changed her intestinal flora that she ultimately accepts as the basis for her ongoing medical concerns. It is as if Sullivan's microbiota serves as a bulwark against her bipolar disorder, and with the colony disrupted through antibiotics, she was no longer protected from the forces that would push her into full-blown bipolar episodes. What followed were several years of depression and mania, during which time she traveled from Australia to Canada, had a severe psychotic episode due to heavy recreational drug use, was hospitalized in a Canadian psychiatric clinic, and eventually returned to Australia. She met her husband-to-be during a relatively "functional" period, and they moved to the Australian outback, where she found some restorative strength in being close to nature.

I was kind of okay, kind of well, and so I moved to the middle of nowhere in rural Australia to live with my husband, and I've been out here seven years. Before the whole poo transplant, gut microbiome stuff, just moving to the bush and spending an inordinate amount of time in nature was very healing, very helpful, and reduced my stress. It was helpful, but I was not functional. I didn't have much of a quality of life and he was really my carer.

Throughout her late teenage years and early adulthood, Sullivan was attended by psychiatrists and other health care providers, who were able to manage her symptoms in limited ways. As she explains, after her eventual diagnosis, the best she could hope for was to not feel suicidal, a state that Sullivan accepts as having "no quality of life." She explains to Parsons that, at the same time she and her partner, Alex, were considering FMT, they were also considering medically-aided death as a result of her extreme psychiatric experiences.

> I believe I was diagnosed in 2011, and my psychiatrist was excellent, and we experimented with a whole lot of different drugs to try and find something that worked. And eventually, we found three drugs that stabilized me to the point where I wasn't suicidal 24 hours a day. But still, I had no quality of life, and I was extremely disabled. I needed to be taken care of by my family, my partner and basically government assistance.

Feeling that this form of life was untenable and willing to risk anything, out of their shared desperation, Sullivan and her partner eventually embarked on their experimental use of FMT. Alex's interest in the procedures was based, at least in part, in his background as an ecologist and reading that he had done on microbiota not as therapeutics, but as part of complex ecosystems. Their willingness to use Alex's feces was due to their understanding that he was a microbial "unicorn," which they explain as similar to the figure of the "super donor." Sullivan recounts that Alex "was born naturally, breastfed, grew up around pets, has been crapped on by a million different types of Australian animals living in the bush, eating with Indigenous people, and anyway, just a really healthy guy who hasn't really experienced stress in his life." She casts Alex as close to nature, from his early life history to his recent interactions with Indigenous people in Australia. This led Sullivan and Alex to their experiment.

> My wonderful husband, because he is an ecologist, he has an understanding of ecosystems and the human body, and the gut microbiome is an ecosystem. Because he reads a lot of journals, he doesn't even re-

member where he came across it, but he read an article in 2016. Actually, the first time he put the idea of a fecal transplant to me was when he read an article about how obesity has shown to be transferable. The fecal matter of an obese person was put into a germ-free mouse, and then they rapidly put on weight and vice versa. And an unfortunate side effect of one of the medications that I was on was rapid weight gain. So before being on this medication I was 60 kilograms. And then within six weeks, I put on 25 kilograms.

The sudden weight gain is the thing that finally tipped Sullivan and Alex toward trying anything out of their desperation for her to become healthy, as they accept the rapid weight gain as a sign of worsening disorder.

We started FMT in November 2016. And really, I was highly skeptical about it, because there was no precedent for doing it for bipolar. I joined all these FMT forums and was asking, has anyone tried this specifically for mental illness, and I couldn't find anyone. We didn't know how often to do it. So basically, we just did one FMT, via enema, every couple of weeks, maybe every two weeks, and at that time, I was severely depressed, like severely depressed, barely able to get out of bed, barely able to even look after my basic hygiene, level of depression. I didn't experience any improvement at all for three months. I don't even know why we kept going. I just kept trying, I guess.... And after about the sixth FMT, and about the three-month mark, something started happening within, and it was like, something started to change. And I remember that my depression just started to subside. It was like this bell curve of the depression starting to get less and less and less and less and less and less. And it was like, Okay, this is actually working, let's do more. And there was a specific day . . . where I woke up and I had this strange feeling that I've never felt before as an adult, and it was like, do I feel good? Is this what feeling good feels like?

As Sullivan notes, there was no indication that FMT could successfully be used for the treatment of bipolar, and how they proceeded was based more on intuition and happenstance than on an established protocol. They muddled into success not through rigorous scientific expertise and testing, but through dogged perseverance—and desperation. Somehow, FMT worked; somehow, Sullivan felt "good."

Conceptualizing how Sullivan becomes "good" depends on opening up the body and exposing the microbial and molecular influences that shape it. The individual human body is popularly understood as a discrete object, bounded by its skin, with its health determined primarily by internal, causal mechanisms, although these may be exacerbated by environmental or lifestyle influences. In order to capture the complexity at work in recent biomedical and scientific paradigms, it is necessary to add two subdermal ways for conceptualizing the body as mentioned in threshold 1: the molecular and the microbial. The first is evident in the interest in genomics and pharmaceuticals, whereas the latter is most clearly demonstrated in medical and scientific attention to the human microbiome. In adding these layers to the body, it becomes apparent how colonization operates at the level of the individual, what its mechanisms are, and how it succeeds and fails. "Colonization" is used by microbiologists, gastroenterologists, patients, and clinicians to describe the process of introducing a "good" microbial community into an unhealthy gut. The molecular body is ruled by discourses about the genetic and epigenetic and moves analysis beyond the bounded, whole body to its biochemical underpinnings; equally important here are industrial chemicals, from pharmaceuticals to hormones, that are accepted as affecting the behaviors and capacities of individual bodies. As such, the molecular body is often perceived as being highly deterministic in its effects and serves as a register for conceptualizing the limits of agentive human powers. The molecular is often accepted as being determinative of our human capacities, particularly at the individual level, where genes or brain chemistry are popularly accepted as shaping the agentive powers of particular people in specific ways, such as the depressed brain, the psychotic brain, or the congenitally disabled.[2]

Beyond the molecular body is the microbial body, comprised of the many nonhuman actors that live on, in, and with human populations. The microbial body is the body as multitude, the individual body as body politic, comprised of a variety of communities of different species that are increasingly accepted by scientists and physicians as shaping the individual and their capacities for digestion, stimulus response, and potentially psychological well-being. Microbial colonies, good and bad, are unruly and difficult to predict, manage, and effectively treat.

Microbial communities are affected by the molecular, and treatments like antibiotics are specifically designed to act on the microbial body, sometimes beneficially by eradicating a bacterial infection, and at other times leading to an imbalance in the microbial body that results in *Clostridium difficile* infection (C. diff.) or similar problems of an unruly colony. The molecular and microbial are accepted by patients, health-care providers, scientists, and nutritionists as having synergistic capacities for changing the individual body, both through molecular therapies and, as in the case of FMT and diet, through microbial ones. Microbial colonies open the question of whether biomedicine's ability to govern the body politic is being significantly challenged in the context of a society that increasingly focuses on the dietary and health benefits of a diverse microbial environment. The molecular and the microbial add smaller scales to conceptualize the body, moving downward in size beyond the encapsulating flesh of the individual body to imperceptible actors inside the body. In scaling down in these ways, the individual becomes less a discrete, skin-contained object, and more a world comprised of microbial populations and molecular forces; they become an ecology intimately connected to the ecology beyond the bounds of the body—a body as landscape. In conceptualizing her body as a landscape, as something connected to its environment through microbial and molecular interactions, Sullivan and her partner recast her symptoms as not a problem of Sullivan's individualized body, but the individual body in relation to its environment. Acting on Sullivan's microbes offers a means to alter the contours of this individualization and rebalance Sullivan's interior conditions and experiences.

Prior to embarking on the FMT experiment, Sullivan consulted her psychiatrist about it, broaching the subject of FMT as therapeutic in general and then as a possible route for her own healing. His responses ranged from the hyperbolic (based on FMT's potential) to the curious:

> I was very hesitant to mention that we were thinking about doing this, but I said, Doctor, you know, what do you think about fecal transplants and bipolar? And he goes, "Jane, it's the medicine of the future. In 20 years, I'll be out of a job, they'll be able to analyze your

gut microbiome and see what species you have missing and give you a tailored probiotic. And all your symptoms will go away. Why do you ask?" I was like, well, we're thinking about trying fecal transplant for my bipolar symptoms, and there was a bit of a pause. And then he was like, well, I'll very interested to see how that turns out.

Sullivan goes on to explain that, after her successful treatment through FMT, she returned to her psychiatrist to tell him about it. Sullivan tells Parsons that, "if [her psychiatrist] hadn't witnessed it himself, he probably wouldn't have believed it. It's an incurable illness, you don't recover. It's unprecedented that I have been in remission for as long as I had, especially not being on medication. It just doesn't happen. Which is why I continue to say that I've cured it." That Sullivan can claim that she is cured is based on both her cessation of symptoms and her constant access to the source of her cure—which could change at any time. Alex's microbiome could change through illness, or he could be injured, or die. Parsons implores Sullivan to freeze some of Alex's feces out of these fears, a suggestion Sullivan takes seriously even if she understands that the efficacy of the FMT samples will decay over time, leaving her without the supplements to her microbiome that have proven so effective. The cure, they all recognize, is a precarious one and one that might slip away.

Whatever uncertainty about FMT exists, disgust remains a critical element in its individual and social acceptance, which Parsons and Sullivan approach in their discussion of Sullivan's later use of capsules to create consumable FMT supplements.

> I learned how to make enteric coated, double encapsulated pills. So I thought, maybe it's a different and maybe [if] the poo goes through the whole digestive tract, it'll colonize other areas. So I did top down method, and it definitely helped. I felt a difference. And so now my sisters want to do pills as well. And I think my mom as well. I mean, I think, psychologically it's a bit more palatable to just swallow pills that look like supplements then an enema.

Parsons responds by saying, "Yeah, not for me. I assume you double encapsulate them to make them clean? You pretty much just do the one that may be messy, but then you put it inside another one?," to which Sullivan goes on to explain how she places the FMT sample into a pill casing, and then, because "you can kind of see the poo in it," she places that capsule inside of another capsule, rendering it more opaque and making the nature of the supplement invisible, at least to those who do not know what it contains. Even Parsons, a dedicated advocate of FMT, has a problem confronting the "ick factor" of orally consuming feces. As discussed in chapter 5, there are efforts to standardize supplements like the one's Sullivan makes, sourced from donors with healthy guts. But it is and always will be someone else's excrement, however curative it might be. Parsons feels like she could not do it ("not for me," she claims), but could it be for you? What would it take to overcome disgust and make the consumption of another person's feces a viable, if not desirable, course of action? What kind of desperation would you need to feel in order to overcome that disgust? This disgust is concretized in institutional conceptions of medicine and its powers, of what counts as medicine and what does not, and this is the terrain on which advocacy for FMT develops in the early twenty-first century, as demonstrated in public and governmental debates about its benefits and risks.

Parsons' disgust is a curious thing. As open as she is to FMT, what she objects to is Sullivan's use of encapsulated fecal samples. Sullivan brings with her a different disgust, informed by her life history and her experiences in and out of Australia; as surely as American disgust comes in specific forms, so too does Australian disgust. But whether consuming FMT capsules sits neatly inside of that regime of disgust is unclear; it is clear, however, that Sullivan acted out of desperation in order to first adopt FMT and then to continue to experiment with it. In confronting Sullivan's practices, Parsons is provided with an opportunity to unsettle her disgust. The outcome of that unsettling process is unclear. But it is grounded in American attitudes toward the body and its porousness that have developed over the course of the twentieth century and provide the foundations for conceptualizing FMT and its dangers.

# 6 Being Gutless
## RACE, KINSHIP, AND MICROBIAL MEDICINE

THE FECAL MICROBIAL TRANSPLANT (FMT) COMMUNITY exists primarily online through patient support groups, many hosted on Facebook or facilitated by websites hosted by clinics or individual wellness coaches. Since 2012, the FMT Friends discussion group has been one of the largest communities,[1] having shared administrative personnel with The Power of Poop, a long-standing, Australia-based website that has promoted the use of FMT through patient narratives and a collection of published scientific articles. Despite its claim of some three thousand members, the active rolls of the FMT Friends community fluctuate, explained by many in the community as a result of people getting better and spending less time in front of their computer and no longer needing community support. Individuals come to the community to ask questions of lay experts and a handful of medical professionals. At any given point in time, a small, active community fields questions from new members as well as returning users. Participants often offer a brief synopsis of their current physiological experience, and then turn to both general and specific questions for the group. One recurrent set of questions focuses on donors. Who makes a good or bad donor, and what are the dangers associated with transplantation? In this respect, the following post from Lucy is exemplary of the genre:

> Such a basic sounding question . . . but how are people finding donors? I understand some has to be through talking to family and friends and links go out and they may be able to find someone that way, but . . . Any other ways? It seems almost hopeless and incredibly rare to find someone healthy enough and it seems that some people are just deciding to do the best they can and use a "healthy enough donor" there

is so much discussion on optimal donors but at this point in history I don't know if there is such a thing and if they are, it's a one in 1 million chance.[2]

Members of the community respond to Lucy by suggesting she turn to members of her family. Her response, which again is typical, runs as follows: "Oh . . . if I had family and friends healthy enough I would have already trialed [the process of testing feces]. So many have been c-section babies and no breastmilk or no breastfeeding at all and histories of courses of antibiotics." FMT seekers are caught between families that are potentially too sick to be able to contribute to their health and the medical-industrial complex that bars them from access to FMT, having restricted it to specific kinds of hospitals and clinics and requiring a willing health-care provider to administer it. At the same time as medical practice in the United States is viewed as the cause of the problems that have led people to seek out FMT as a therapy, it is also seen as the possible source of a solution, if the U.S. government finally permits widespread use of FMT and health-care providers overcome the "ick factor." As discussed in chapter 5, the problem that the Food and Drug Administration has identified is the current state of unknowability about what precisely is in the samples that donors provide and what effect, if any, it might have on the recipients of FMT procedures. When successful, FMT has exquisite effects; but what might FMT convey along with that curative? This question has led scientists and physicians to fear that hepatitis, type 2 diabetes, obesity, and potentially neurological disorders might be transmitted through FMT. The challenge is an empirical one, shaped by contemporary understandings of the microbiome, technologies used to assess it, and the relationship between diseases and microbial colonies.

Half-jokingly, the members of the FMT online community refer to themselves as "pooineers," indexing their role as experimental guinea pigs in the controversial landscape of microbial medicine. At the same time as they are asked to reconceptualize their kinship network not as based on the typical forms of biological and legal reckoning that position some people as kin and others as not, but rather as "good" and "bad" donors based on questions of health, diet, chronic illness, antibiotic exposure, and histories of mental illness; they are also tasked with reworking their relationship to the state, primarily through their engagement with medical institutions, and specifically research hospitals who have filed applications with the FDA for the use of FMT in the case of *Clostridium difficile* (C. diff.) infections. But the experimental status of FMT also drives patients to peri-legal, informal networks of feces donors, internet support groups, and online resources, where government regulation meets its limits and instead depends on self-regulation through disgust.

I take this position as "pooineers" seriously, focusing on the ideal medical practices that FMT seekers are striving to experience, while also attending to how they are asked to fall back on their kinship networks as resources in the face of uneven and unpredictable medical access and care. In recomposing one's kinship network, unlikely qualities of personhood and microbial stewardship come into play: As mentioned in the above Facebook post, questions about antibiotic use, vaginal birth, breastfeeding, diet, and personal histories of illness and well-being all become germane to considering who makes an appropriate donor and who makes "good" kin. In ruling individuals out of donorship, one reworks the contours of a kinship network, seeking to become more like those with healthy microbiomes and less like those—often reproductive-biological kin— who are unhealthy. The figures of the "ideal donor" and "super donor" loom large in producing aspirational desires for FMT seekers, but they are more likely to have to fall back on donors who are "healthy enough." The "pooineer" is compelled to explore a terrain of risk and exposure. This exploration is motivated by medical desperation, with individuals driven to experiment with potentially dangerous self-administered treatments, which serves to compose the contours of emerging forms of American kinship.

Here, I approach kinship as a conduit. Traditionally, anthropologists conceptualize kinship as a kind of relation, with one's status as kin being either positive or negative: one is either related to someone else or is not. Over time, anthropologists have argued that kinship is a cultural system of relations and should not be reduced to mere biological understandings of relatedness.[3] As a cultural system, it often makes recourse to biological tropes, utilizing "blood" and "genes" as ways to reckon relatedness between individuals and families, as well as racialized and ethnic communities. Conceptualizing kinship as a conduit asks not whether one person is related to another person, but what that principle relation opens up in terms of extended relations. Kinship-as-conduit demonstrates what people are willing to be related to and what they are not. This is predicated on the understanding of the body as permeable, as changeable through the process of FMT and other microbial medicines, and this conception is compounded by assumptions about race embedded in discussions of diet, disease, dirt, and disgust. Attitudes about not-relating overlap materialist understandings of the world, and bodies within it, and serve as a cultural screen against relatedness. This is vital in the context of the turn toward microbial conceptions of human life, where microbial actors are recognized as determining gut health, undercutting human-to-human forms of relatedness by acknowledging microbial agents and their agencies. As the May 2013 workshop held by the FDA and the National Institutes of Health (NIH) attests, microbial actors are accepted as potential vectors of illness, many of which are understood in racial terms and in the context of the racialized stratification of health and well-being in the United States.

The surge of microbial medicine in the early 2000s, particularly in the context of American consumerist biomedicine, forces attention onto the relationship among microbes, conceptions of race, and racial anxieties. But doing so depends on moving beyond static understandings of race and racism that reify phenotypic understandings of race while they seek to dismantle them; instead, I focus here on the implicit (and sometimes explicit) ways that the science and medicine of FMT get enrolled into racist political structures. The construction of the process of FMT as neutral and transparent allows it to carry both the feces of FMT and the shit of racism. Making this move depends on comprehending that the microbial is inherently associated with race, and that what a turn to the microbial accomplishes is providing a screen that allows medical science to operate in a seemingly postracial space where the race of a donor is ostensibly unimportant. This allows race to become associated with particular capacities, evident here in susceptibilities to specific diseases and abilities to eat and digest particular foods. As a result, race is read into microbes, reflected most clearly in discussions about the suitability of raced bodies to be FMT donors, a move that takes the implicit and makes it explicit. FMT makes new kin possible and renders new understandings of kinship apparent, and it is precisely because of these potentials that questions of donorship become important to practitioners and FMT seekers.

In the following, I begin by working through the figures of the "ideal" and "super" donor. I then turn to discussions of the donors individuals have access to, many of whom are only "good enough" and nowhere near the standards set by medical science. This failure on the part of kin to meet these clinical standards compels interventions on the part of those who would be in receipt of their microbial transfusions to make them into better, if not ideal, donors. These negotiations stand against a backdrop of the racial understanding of health in the United States and elsewhere, with some kinds of people being more exposed to illness than others. Certain kinds of people are de facto "bad" donors because of their diets, environmental exposures, and hereditary lines. These disqualifying attributes are associated, implicitly and sometimes explicitly, with racialized categories. In this way, the explorations of these "pooineers," most of whom are white, is conducted on a terrain of racial disparities and racist sentiment. I then turn to recent trends in dieting that aim to provide the foundation for stewarding one's microbial colony by feeding it on, or in some cases starving it of, specific foods, trends that provide a purposeful practice that guides microbe-focused eaters as they experiment with the colony within, extending a century of dietary self-regulation from John Harvey Kellogg and Adelle Davis through the present. I conclude by returning to the questions of race, racism, kinship, and microbial medicine and its potentials.

## Ideal and Super Donors

In their development of the protocol for the Fecal Microbiota Transplant National Registry, Gary Wu, Loren Laine, and Colleen Kelly relied on the American Association of Blood Bank's donor questionnaire. Anyone who has donated blood in the United States would recognize most of the questions and might specifically remember the questions pertaining to intravenous drug use and prostitution, both of which are accepted as flags for hepatitis and HIV/AIDS. Beyond this set of questions meant to assess one's risk of blood-borne infections, the FMT questionnaire seeks to assess one's exposure to antibiotics and experiences that are accepted as disrupting microbial balance. As a document, it enacts forms of medical racism that construct particular kinds of donors as impossible donors, while others, known through absences of disqualifying features, become normal donors. Ideal and super donors exceed these expectations in ways that are difficult to quantify and instead trade on culturally valued characteristics, if not actual capacities or qualities.

The questionnaire asks specifically about periods of time spent in the United Kingdom during the period in which mad cow disease was of concern, and generally about time spent in Europe adding up to a total of five years or time spent in the military. It also specifically asks whether the donor has "had sexual contact with anyone who was born or lived in Africa" or "been in Africa." There is no mention of any other part of the Global South, no mention of South or Central America or South Asia. Only Africa is named—and named as a whole continent. These questions are sandwiched between one that asks whether the respondent has ever "had any type of cancer (including leukemia)"or "had sex for drugs or money." It is worth noting that this is the second time that a question about the respondent's own possible prostitution occurs, and there is a third when one includes the question asking whether the respondent has had sex with someone who has engaged in prostitution. Coupled with the question regarding one's cancer history, these geographic questions, and especially the questions about Africa, should be read as being about a contaminating exposure that an individual has experienced. Whereas the questions regarding time spent in Europe and the United Kingdom are temporally limited ("From 1980 to the present"), the questions regarding Africa are framed as "Have you *ever* . . . ?" One might counter that particular pathogens are found only in Africa, but this elides the fact that Africa is enormous and diverse, and such a general question obscures more than it reveals about donor histories. What it does clearly reveal is the symbolic weight "Africa" holds in the American medical imagination and how it threatens to contaminate individual donor histories; the questions build an association between Africa and dangerous excrement.

The shadow cast by these questions implies an ideal donor. Gender and sex do not seem to matter to one's status as a stool donor, yet a donor should have not been exposed to antibiotics within the last six months, but ideally much longer; they should not have a current infection of any sort, nor be treating a recent infection. They should not have used intravenous drugs, eaten meat infected with mad cow, had a blood transfusion or received an organ transplant or bone graft, or been exposed to hepatitis. They should not have any diseases currently associated with the gut, including irritable bowel syndrome, Crohn's, ulcerative colitis, chronic diarrhea, gastrointestinal cancers, and celiac disease. They should not have used human growth hormone, be related to anyone with Creutzfeldt-Jakob disease, have any autoimmune disorders, or "neurological diseases" including Parkinson's, autism, or ALS. They should not have been in jail or prison for more than three days, in Europe for longer than five years, or in Africa, "ever."

In many cases, these expectations are reasonable and based on doubts in contemporary medical science. Can diabetes be transmitted via FMT? No one is entirely sure, but it is unlikely. Can hepatitis or any other bloodborne disease? Again, it is unclear, but probably not. Can neurological disorders? Without extensive research, that too will remain in doubt. It is especially difficult with regards to neurological disorders precisely because FMT is currently being experimented with to cure neurological conditions, or to at least minimize their symptoms, including Alzheimer's and autism. If a healthy colony can cure or minimize these disorders, can a bad colony cause or exacerbate them? These implicit racialized fears find traction in epidemiological data that shows disease prevalence among nonwhites is higher than among whites. Epidemiological research shows, repeatedly, that non-Hispanic whites have the lowest rate of diabetes, while non-Hispanic Blacks are only behind Native Americans and Alaskan Natives in terms of diabetes rates.[4] Across its three types, A, B, and C, hepatitis is associated with poverty and nonwhite immigrants to the United States. Recently, rates among the rural poor, especially white rural poor, have increased as a side effect of widespread intravenous drug use associated with opiates.[5] Mortality rates across hepatitis infections are higher among nonwhites than white people. This follows general epidemiological rates among nonwhite populations in the United States, who are more likely both to be exposed to disease-causing sources and to die of complications associated with disease as a result of structural inequalities. Race as a proxy for illness exposure makes sense given epidemiological data, but it obscures the political contexts in which exposure is differentially produced.[6]

If it is too strong of a claim to say that the ideal donor is white, it is clear that the qualities associated with the ideal donor are those associated with a particular form of American whiteness. The ideal donor is expected to have exempted themselves from travel, restricted sexual activity, avoided illegal drugs, and had a clear understanding of those in their social world and their backgrounds. Exposures to geographical places, with their racialized associations and kinds of practices and people serve as proxies to assess the racialized capacities of a potential donor. The ideal donor is transparent and without qualities, and in this neutral abstraction is accepted as having a potentially powerful microbial colony for the purpose of FMT. The super donor, on the other hand, has very specific qualities, serving as the realization of historical and contemporary processes of stewardship that have resulted in a superior microbial colony.

In 2018, reports began to circulate about "super donors," those individuals with microbiomes that behaved in particularly exquisite ways, with greater efficacy than modal donors. The term "super donor" was concretized by Brooke Wilson, Tommi Vatanen, Wayne Cutfield, and Justin O'Sullivan in their publication of "The Super-Donor Phenomenon in Fecal Microbiota Transplantation."[7] Ironically, they sought to overturn the very idea of the super donor, seeking to upset the "one stool fits all" approach in gastroenterology. The assumption buried in "one stool fits all" is that one superior set of qualities could be ascertained, and those donors could be relied on for providing samples to cure all complaints that FMT might target, much like Lee Jones, CEO of Rebiotix, expressed interest in doing in chapter 5. Instead, in their meta-analysis of the existing literature, Wilson and her coauthors propose that a more precise approach is mandated: "It appears that the most important factors predicting strain engraftment in FMT are taxonomic identity and strain abundance in both the donor and the recipient prior to FMT."[8] This suggests that what is required for a successful match between donor and recipient is a careful selection of sympathetic relationships between donor microbiota and what the recipient lacks. The implication of this is that difference between the donor and recipient is mandated, and that similarity—as biological kinship might presume—is ruled out.

In lieu of an actual "super donor," Wilson and company suggest that a precise match between donor and recipient is necessary to provide therapeutic effects.

> It appears a patient's response to FMT predominantly depends on the capability of the donor's microbiota to restore the specific metabolic disturbances associated with their particular disease phenotype. If this is true, a donor-recipient matching approach, where a patient is screened to identify the functional perturbations specific to their microbiome, may be the best way forward. The patient could then be matched to a specific FMT donor known to be enriched in taxa associated with the metabolic pathway that needs to be restored.[9]

The infrastructure required to make these matches does not currently exist, and what pieces of it do exist are insufficient to fully screen potential donors and match them to waiting recipients. As they address throughout their review, it is also unclear exactly which microbial strains benefit each complaint that FMT is currently used for, meaning that matching a potential treatment to an unknown disorder exceeds current medical science. Rather than a super donor, Wilson and her coauthors suggest that there are some donors who are better donors than others, precisely because their microbial colonies are more diverse: "High diversity of the gut microbiota, particularly in the donor, appears to best predict a patient's response to FMT. More specifically, the efficacy of FMT likely depends on the ability of the donor to provide the necessary taxa capable of restoring metabolic deficits in recipients that are contributing toward disease."[10] This call for "high diversity" implicitly suggests that the super donor might still be possible to identify, but that in the super donor's absence, being able to identify donors with highly diverse microbial communities might serve the same ends, albeit without a clear understanding of how their effectiveness is achieved.

Super donors, as well as ideal donors, raise questions about the milieu in which donors live. What are their diets? What are their medical histories? Were they breastfed, and birthed vaginally? These questions are important precisely because their answers seem to index the bases for optimal microbial health. The challenge with these questions is that they operate on two temporal scales. The first is the everyday, where questions about daily practice, specifically related to diet, seem to provide answers to why an ideal donor's microbiome contains certain loads of particular bacteria, both positive and negative. Wheat and sugar are the most likely perceived threats, and individuals with diverse, probiotic diets are accepted as better stewards of their microbiome than those with narrow diets or those who rely on too much prepared food. With the aid of diets, microbiomes can be altered, and specific diets have been developed to curate to beneficial microbes and starve pernicious ones—or at least that is what they are imagined to be doing.

The second temporal scale is that of an individual's lifetime, literally starting at birth. The dominant view is that one's microbial community is established at birth, with vaginal birth bestowing on an individual the essential microbial communities of one's mother.[11] In addition, being breastfed is accepted as helping to develop that microbial community, and individuals who were formula-fed and delivered via cesarean section are rated as less than optimal donors. Contemporary diet decisions are overlaid on these foundations, and individuals who have healthy diets and limited environmental exposures are accepted as potentially overcoming the disadvantages of their early life. Both of these temporal scales, the everyday and the lifetime, become associated with race. The first maps onto everyday exposures, from urban landscapes to everyday diets, that rule individuals out of being ideal or super donors. The second maps onto perceptions of childrearing and the realities of maternal care in the U.S. medical industry, with nonwhites being less likely to breastfeed.[12] In both cases, race serves as a proxy for an individual's exposures, with nonwhite bodies being accepted as more risky than white ones. A similar logic appears in FMT seeker attitudes toward donation, apparent in Facebook-support-group conversations.

## "Pioneer Science Shit"

Reporting on her experience with FMT, Facebook-group member Rebecca says: "It is different for everyone. I had cramping, fatigue, low energy, weight gain, and body aches immediately after the FMT. The energy never returned to pre-FMT normal and my weight continues to increase. (Until the FMT I was energetic and thin). Other people have had success.

Unfortunately, I wasn't one of them." Picking up on Rebecca's discussion of weight gain, another commenter, Jack, who is a medical researcher asks: "You had an overweight donor, didn't you?" The dialogue continues: "It turns out I did. I was told she was 'normal body weight' (not true). Now I deal with feeling like I am living with someone else's sluggish overweight body stuck in mine." It is unclear whether Rebecca's donor was in fact overweight; she should have no way of knowing, since the clinic should not disclose this information. But in this interchange, the weight status of her donor is quickly ratified against the assumption that her "energetic and thin" status was not the byproduct of her illness, but her natural state. In her antifat perspective, that natural state is colonized by the "sluggish overweight body" that the FMT procedure sympathetically contaminates her with, making her less her pre-illness self, and more akin to her unknown donor.

Jack assures her, however, that the sympathetic process can occur in reverse: "You can reverse those symptoms finding a slender donor with a very clean medical history, no history of being overweight, and a clean diet. Someone active. And if a medical clinic did this to you and lied about their donor, you might consider a lawsuit." Rebecca replies: "A medical clinic did the FMT. It can be reversed?! That would be amazing! How would I eliminate the biome from the first donor to replace it with someone new?" Jack replies:

> Yeah, it "can" be reversed. Theoretically. We do it in mice models all day long. Make fat ones skinny and skinny ones fat by fecal transplants. The same thing happens with our own microbiomes. It doesn't mean you won't just introduce new side-effects, however. This is not even close to a perfected science. This is pioneer science shit. It's all about finding the right donor "for you."

What is being negotiated here are the "natural" states of bodies and how, through superimposition through FMT, these natures become colonized. The science of FMT, at least for Jack, is both "pioneer science shit" and also a process that operates in a transparently sympathetic, colonizing way. While there may be doubts about the science, which Jack captures in his invocation of "pioneer science shit," FMT is also accepted unproblematically as the mechanism through which Rebecca went from being "energetic and thin" to "sluggish" and "overweight." Jack goes on to suggest that "it's all about finding the right donor 'for you,'" implying that the "right" kind of donor is one that shares a natural, pre-illness state with the recipient. As much as these natural states are perceived as being indebted to one's birth, one's early diet, and one's genetics, they are also shaped by one's exposure to antibiotics, contemporary diet, and everyday life. His suggestion is that Rebecca's contemporary condition is the result of using the wrong donor, not the result of an unpredictable procedure or her everyday life.

Jack goes on to suggest that the real danger is more widespread colonialism: "If they are using overweight people as donors for you, they're doing it [to] other people too. That same overweight, sluggish donor probably donated several samples they are using on patients currently." Rebecca, in this figuration, is a bellwether case, the first obvious example of the contamination of a population of patients with the wrong kind of donor. Rebecca's implication is that the clinic knew the status of her donor as "sluggish" and "overweight" and used the samples anyway, thereby facilitating this process of colonial contamination. Jack's invocation of the law and the need to stop this colonization process is due to his surety that the same clinic is affecting "other people too," and likely that lax oversight and screening processes are allowing other bad colonies to sympathetically contaminate an unwitting and desperate population. From there, the threat is that these bad colonies compel a cascading descent into sickness for their recipients, who, in their desperation, trade one disordered state of being for another.

Pooineership and "pioneer science shit" are both predicated on the emergent conception of the human body as the medium for microbial colonies. At once, they rely on both an understanding of the natural status of pre-illness bodies and the possibility that a human body can be a neutral vessel, devoid of an existing colony, and an able, if not always willing, recipient of a donor colony. The problems, then, are a recipient's ability to be changed by a donor's colony, the danger that bad donor colonies will come to contaminate unwitting recipients, and that the "right" donors cannot be identified. The neutral conduit of the body brings people together in unexpected and potentially dangerous ways. They become united not through blood or law, but through microbial contamination.

This sympathetic kinship between bodies, beneficial and detrimental, threatens dominant conceptions of kinship as based in blood and law, and replaces them with a conception of the microbial, biological connection between bodies. It also works against the unsympathetic tendencies in American biomedicine. The threat is that dangerous colonies will contaminate already ill bodies, compounding their disordered state. The threat is also that this sympathetic kinship will bring bodies into relation in undesirable and unpredictable ways. Being gutless—the very status that allows one to be healed—also opens up visceral connections through the unknown and unknowable.

## Racial Permeability

"I'm wondering if it's okay to do FMT with a donor of another race?" So begins a post from Theodore. He goes on: "As I live in Japan, my options are limited to Japanese people. However, being Scottish, I wonder if there are any known issues about using a donor from a completely different race? I have had [ulcerative colitis; IBD] for five years." Theodore goes on to explain that he has "read that there is something in the Japanese gut that helps with the digestion (?) of seaweed that we don't have." It is unclear how Theodore understands race, or the relationship between race and diet. But he implies that there is an integral connection that allows Japanese people to digest their diet in ways that Scottish, and presumably white people more generally, cannot. Whatever assumptions about race Theodore holds, they are largely ratified by the group as they negotiate the benefits of crossracial donation. Race, they posit, is isomorphic with diet; and yet dietary capacity and microbial colony are transferrable through the process of FMT. If there are dangers, at least in Theodore's initial query, they seem to amount to little more than the possibility that something might ease his digestion of seaweed. The conversation that this inquiry spawns, however, ranges across concerns with racial permeability, the relationship between diet and environment, and the association of specific parts of the world with exposure to "dirt" and (potentially) beneficial microbial communities.

Considering microbial transfers encourages conceptualizing race differently. Rather than the phenotypic understanding of race (that skin, hair, or other obvious physical features constitute one's racial know-ability), examining how racial anxieties adhere to the seemingly neutral process of FMT focuses attention on how racial capacities might be transferred between bodies. Race, in this model, is less a molar, whole-bodied feature, and more a discrete physiological capacity, captured in the above-mentioned "something in the Japanese gut that helps with the digestion (?) of seaweed." The permeability of bodies might be posited as a source of racial anxiety; one can become "Japanese" or (as I discuss below) "Kenyan" through the process of FMT in a way that typical conceptions of race normally disallow, but which echo ideas about race from Kellogg, Davis, and Weston Price.

The conversation that emerges from Theodore's initial query moves in two directions. The first focuses on the relationship between racial capacities and microbial colonies. The second focuses on the relationship between cultural environments, especially concerns with "dirt," and how they shape the bodies that exist within them. Taken together, these conceptions of diet, environment, cultural practice, and microbial powers suggest that race is transmissible, much like the screening procedures in FMT donation. This transmission is not phenotypic, but related to racial capacities. The anxiety that provokes questions like Theodore's is precisely this: racial capacities are accepted as facilitated through the neutral process of FMT, enacting a potential colonization in reverse, white bodies becoming less white through FMT. The challenge, as the conversation allows, is that in this case racial mixing, or wholesale crossbody colonization, might be beneficial.

In this respect, consider Erin's response to Theodore's query:

> Well it might actually be beneficial for you. If you have IBD and are Anglo celtic—as I am also, there's plenty of evidence on pubmed to suggest that we have an ethnic susceptibility to the disease. This however is not the case with Asians—who are much less likely to develop IBD. So maybe having bacteria from a Japanese will actually place you in a superior position.

For Erin, "ethnic susceptibility" indexes her understanding of racial capacities. Despite her use of "ethnicity" here, Erin is ascribing this difference in microbial colonies to Asians in general. Her conflation of race and ethnicity provides her with the ability to differentiate "Anglo Celtics" from "Asians," and "Japanese" in particular, and to suggest that the possibility of supplementing Theodore's IBD-prone microbial disposition with an Asian infusion would place him in a superior position to other "Anglo Celtics." A similar view is held by Stanley, who accepts microbial capacities as simultaneously linked to local environments and yet in need of changing when one changes environments.

> I'm of the view that a healthy Asian microbiome would be good for me while in asia (im in China) if I went the FMT path. It's the part when I return to Australia that I'm not sure about. Theodore, my Crohns has improved markedly after living in China 6 years (where everything is a little more dirty and the food a little more natural), and every time I go back to Australia I get rashes and allergies popping up. Don't know what to put it down to though. It's all very fascinating yet frustrating.

Stanley's reporting on his experience in China and its curative effects on his gut inspires a response from Erin, who similarly was born in Australia and found herself living in China. "I lived in China for several years and went into complete remission there—only getting sick upon returning to Australia. Go figure?" Stanley asks Erin what she puts her "remission in China down to," to which she responds: "I think it might have been lots of vegetables and very little red meat, no dairy and no wheat. Also litres of tea—which is an antibacterial! And stacks of bacteria probably . . . well as you know . . . China is not the cleanest of places."

At stake in Erin and Stanley's interchange is the kinship between microbes, people, and their environments. In the case of their environments, Stanley and Erin accept the body as porous, both responding to natural cues—as in Stanley's fear of a return to Australia and the effects it will have on his body—and dietary influences. Stanley and Erin share an association between China and "dirt" demonstrated in Stanley's invocation of China being "where everything is a little more dirty and the food a little more natural" and Erin's "China is not the cleanest of places." These environmental influences are superimposed onto the natural state of the body, explicit in Erin's use of "Anglo Celtic" to describe the physiological susceptibility of specific individuals to IBD. This same assumption undergirds Stanley's understanding that his body is mismatched with the environment of Australia and is reflected in the screening of FMT donors and the use of geographical exposures as a proxy for disease susceptibility.

The same set of kinship concerns about bodies, permeability, and environments is demonstrated in the other responses that Theodore's query elicits from the community. They fall along similar lines of reasoning, divided between those who anticipate dangers associated with using samples from a "different race" and those who accept potential benefits from the marriage between microbial colonies. For example, Stacy writes: "Personally I think the more diversity the better. Our weakened Western microbiomes are causing a lot [of] health problems," which is juxtaposed to Karen's claim that "I personally would not cuz I had a reaction to someone of different race BUT I heard other people have success." Similarly, Peter writes: "My personal view is its generally more risky especially using donor who may have been exposed to more harmful bacteria in their lifetime than your system might have—they may still be a carrier and/or have a genetic disposition to handle their biome whereas another race may not." Finally, Sherman suggests that "I think that Hybrid Vigor is essential for any living thing. If your donor, irrespective of where they come from, has a clean pathology test, I would suggest Go for It, Lucky You!" Across these conversational interventions, race is both accepted as being associated with place and deemed irrelevant; race is accepted as a marker of one's riskiness, with more dangerous donors associated (with race as a proxy) with particular places, family histories, cultural practices, and diets. There is no resolution to a shared conception of race. What is accepted is the assumption that FMT will convey, unproblematically, the microbial capacities of one body to another. There may be synergistic benefits; there are also, as Peter notes, "risks" that adhere to crossrace donation, predicated on kinship between bodies facilitated by FMT.

In this context of suspicion and understanding of racial permeability, consider the interchange between Vinay, a South Asian man in India, and Noah, a white man in the United States:

> I am from India and i am considering FMT, My issue is that i have lost my appetite, i lost almost 15 kg weight in 2 months four years back and not yet gained or loose anymore. My immunity is lower than

before and my stool consistency is also very crapped, its solid, soft and liquid at same time. . . . I am friend with a Kenyan person and he lives in my city, he seems like a good donor because these people are generally more healthier than us, What could be side effects of using the poop of a different race person, he is 2–3 inch taller than me and built wise he has athletic body.

Vinay's conception of race appears to be more reductive than Erin's, Stanley's, and Theodore's, associated strictly with phenotypic qualities and captured in his use of "these people" and the focus on the size of the "Kenyan person" and their "athletic body." Noah responds to Vinay's conception of race by dissuading Vinay's concern with race and invoking their shared status as pooineers in relation to the "uncharted territory" that FMT use represents.

I personally wouldn't assume anything. IMO, race is irrelevant. As long as you do proper testing and the donor passes the testing, rest of the stuff carries a very little weight. Just FYI, FMT is not a silver bullet, everyone may not benefit. There are a lot of factors involved and I doubt, we know even 10% of them. This is an uncharted territory for majority of us.

Noah's dismissal of race as a question of concern might be read as a specifically postracial appeal. But this is undercut by his suggestion that "we [don't] know even 10%" of the factors involved in FMT. The risks that stem from these doubts are the terrain of pooineership, and Noah's attempt to get Vinay to move beyond phenotypic conceptions of race is an effort to move him toward a microbial conception of race that relies not on molar features of the body, but rather the invisible influences of the colony within.

## Stewarding the Colony Within

In the fall of 2020, amid the Covid-19 pandemic and political tensions in the United States and globally, a series of videos posted to a public Facebook group dedicated to the support of individuals with gastrointestinal disorders garnered a significant amount of interest from its community members. The videos depicted a young man, Peter, sitting outdoors, perched on the edge of a chaise lounge. He is in his early thirties, white, with blonde hair and a few days' beard growth. The first video is largely wordless, and we watch as he pinches his nose and gulps down a shake he has prepared for himself. The shake is a reddish brown, and it is only by reading the comments on the video that one can learn what is in it: a mix of berries, distilled water, and a fecal sample from Peter's girlfriend, to whom he refers as a "high quality donor," all blended to a drinkable viscosity. In thirty seconds, the shake is consumed and he stands up to walk away; all we hear is his off-screen girlfriend say "Wow" as he puts aside the empty glass. This is followed by another video, in which Peter explains that he has cut the fruit out of the shake, leaving only distilled water and feces, resulting in a squarely brown shake that he proceeds to gulp down. A third video is eventually posted, in which Peter is joined by a guest, whom Peter aids in consuming a shake, again provided by Peter's girlfriend. Each is peppered with comments from viewers and Peter's answers to their concerns. Across his answers it is clear that his experiment is motivated by a growing sense that changing one's microbial community is critical to his conception of well-being. Any disgust expressed by his audience is parried away: he insists that feces from a "high quality donor" is less disgusting and easier to swallow. He infers that you too can fix your gut by consuming the right kind of excremental medicine. Moreover, use of FMT can be supplemented by the daily maintenance of the microbiome through diet. This everyday regime of treatment through diet provides individuals with a sense of control over their bodies through the regulations they impose on their everyday forms of food consumption, governed by rules associated with diets that target microbial appetites and the effects of feeding particular microbial actors. In this way, care for one's microbial community scales between the knowable, everyday management of diet and the unknowable and unpredictable horizon of an event-to-come and the resurgence of a chronic illness that FMT attempts to mitigate. In between, through the human–nonhuman relationship of a person and their microbial community, the "flare up" of that chronic illness can be held at bay. Producing an intimacy between an individual and the microbial colony that lies within their body ensures that the colony within is being properly stewarded.

What made Peter's videos of interest to the Facebook community he is a part of is that he drinks the materials that he has prepared for himself. Most at-home users of FMT use a "bottom" method, meaning that they employ an enema to get the material into their colon and small intestine. Using a "top" method—drinking the shake or using a gavage or prepared pills—targets the large intestine, which, as Peter describes, has a much larger surface area and is home to a greater multitude of microbes. In many respects, reaching the large intestine is the Holy Grail of excremental medical treatments, in that it likely has greater effects on human health and, because of patients' discomfort with "top" treatments, is difficult to accomplish. What is often described as the "ick factor" is too much for most FMT users to consider, particularly when "bottom" treatments are largely effective for their complaints.[13] What is also critical in Peter's account is that he comes to cut food out of the shake. Instead, Peter suggests a treatment regime that he refers to as the "Funky 7": a shake followed by seven days of fasting, drinking only distilled water, in an effort to get the newly introduced microbes to focus on establishing themselves by consuming other, more troublesome colony members. This internally focused effort at microbial management is a kind of stewardship, a management of the self through the control of nonhuman others. It is most readily apparent in Peter's fasting, but is also key to several diets that FMT users employ to manage their microbial colonies. Stewardship aims to balance human desires with nonhuman needs, often shaping the effects of nonhuman life in ways that provide positive outcomes for humans. And, critically, stewardship works across scales: it is how the management of the colony within motivates the control of environments and their resources in the world at large for human well-being, and potentially for nonhuman and environmental well-being as well.

Two diets are exemplary here, the GAPS diet ("gut and psychological/physiology syndrome") and the SIBO diet ("small intestine bacterial overgrowth"). Both are restrictive diets in that they seek to regulate what people are eating in order to identify the root causes of medical disorder, which both locate in the gut, and then treat that disorder by restricting the body's consumption of materials that lead to "flare ups" and dysbiosis. Both diets identify a host of environmental and social factors that lead to imbalanced microbial colonies, from the use of pesticides in agriculture and highly processed industrial foodstuff, to the absence of fat in food, to the Standard American Diet, to the importance of vaginal birth and breastfeeding. In making these causal claims, the diet promoters posit that the incidental experiences of individuals are actually the result of long-standing political-economic forces that shape everything from consumer behaviors to parenting practices, which builds on thinkers like Davis and Benjamin Spock and collectively places the onus of change on the individual and their management of their microbial colony. If the physiological effects of these decisions cannot be fundamentally changed, they can be mitigated through stewardship. At its best, stewardship binds the individual to their environment through a widening conception of body–environment interactions and a set of responsibilities to care not only for the self, but for nonhuman others and one's environment. More than just collections of recipes, the cookbooks for these diets offer guides for living that seek to help people conceptualize themselves as porous, dismembered bodies and offer understandings of how bodies and their environments interact as a system. In this way, these diets participate in an ideological project that stretches through American history and connects with liberal, health-centered efforts from Kellogg to the present. Moreover, they seek to make the individual one who is charged with their own stewardship responsibilities, independent from the dangers that are associated with FMT and the transmissibility of racialized capacities.

The small intestinal bacterial overgrowth from which the acronym SIBO comes is a condition in which the bacterial community in the small intestine is imbalanced, often leading to malabsorption of nutrients. Sylvie McCracken, author of *The SIBO Solution* describes the problem in this way:

> When you have too much bacteria in your gut, the bacteria will start feeding off of undigested particles of food. The bacteria causes the starches to ferment. The fermentation process produces hydrogen gas as a byproduct. If you have an overgrowth of bacteria, then the bacteria are going to have a field day eating away at your food—before your body can even start digesting them. You end up with a gut full of hydrogen gas. With the methane-producing type of SIBO, . . . there is also an over-growth of archaea, which are single-cell organisms with-

out a nucleus. The archaea feed off of hydrogen, but they produce methane as a byproduct. In either case, you end up with a lot of gas in your gut.[14]

The goal of the SIBO diet is to identify which bacteria are causing problems for an individual through a restriction of the kinds of nutrients and foodstuffs that particular bacteria consume. The result is weeding out sugars and carbohydrates, both of which result in intestinal fermentation. It also includes cutting out food that is fermented. This means a diet that is inclusive of meats but not their processed counterparts; small amounts of most vegetables, but no onions or garlic or anything starchy, like potatoes, or acidic, like tomatoes; berries and bananas, but not apples and stone fruits; small amounts of nuts, coffee, alcohol, and juice; cultured dairy, but nothing processed; animal fats, but no seed oils or margarine.[15] The challenge that McCracken identifies is that the Standard American Diet relies on simple carbohydrates, sugars, processed meats and dairy, and sugary fruits, all of which feed bacteria in ways that result in continued poor health for the humans involved. The individual is then put in the position of needing to square their desires, expectations of health, and sense of microbial needs. Because this kind of treatment is extraclinical, the costs—both financial and temporal—are borne by an individual and their family. This can be considerable, particularly when the assumptions underlying much of the foodstuff that makes up this diet is meant to be organic, unpasteurized, and unprocessed. It can also be challenging to overcome eaters' expectations of what counts as desirable food, particularly when many of the foods that the SIBO diet endorses are less processed and more "natural" than those around which the Standard American Diet is built.

In many respects, the SIBO diet is similar to the GAPS diet, which was first designed by Natasha Campbell-McBride.[16] As GAPS can stand for both "gut and *psychology* syndrome" and "gut and *physiology* syndrome," it can include everything from gut-related digestive concerns to autism, schizophrenia, and ADHD (attention-deficit/hyperactivity disorder). The GAPS diet is predicated on the assumption that our modern diets are the cause of our medical disorders, and that, like paleo diets,[17] a return to "ancestral" dietary practices will improve our health by restoring gut microbes to something akin to that of imagined human ancestors.[18] This involves, much like the SIBO diet, a strong reliance on fatty foods, with meat, dairy, and nuts holding a pride of place. What is left out, without exception, are grains, sugars, starchy vegetables, starchy legumes, and lactose. Because what GAPS seeks to treat is so diverse, with likewise diverse causes, the diet's execution is largely individual. Mary Brackett, one of the authors of the GAPS-influenced *The Heal Your Gut Cookbook* points out: "I learned that although a food might be nourishing for one person, it could be damaging to another. After years of being told to 'listen to your doctor' for answers, it took me a while to listen to my own body to determine what was actually my medicine and my poison."[19] What is consistent across individual executions of the diet, according to Campbell-McBride, is that it is meant to be based on "Nature." She writes: "When Mother Nature made us humans, she at the same time provided us with every food we need to stay healthy, active and full of energy. . . . Natural foods get changed into various chemical concoctions, which are then packaged nicely and presented to us as 'food.'"[20] Embracing the GAPS diet is an attempt to align microbial health with individual health, and both with the health of the environment, captured in Campbell-McBride's use of "Mother Nature." For example, an embrace of organic, biodynamic foods aims to restore both the environment and its ecosystem and the human as a part of that ecosystem. "Food" and the artificial stand in opposition to these efforts, necessitating a form of care that unifies approaches to the self, the nonhuman, and the environmental.

How chronic illness is conceptualized often depends on ideas about care for the self and care for the human other. These forms of care are supported by and motivated through institutions that aim to support both the cared for and the carers.[21] But microbial medicine, and particularly excremental medicine, draws attention to the need to care for the nonhuman environments both inside and outside of our bodies. Fundamental here are conceptions of the permeability of the body and the need to manage the interior of the body through the ingestion of food—or in the case of Peter's "Funky 7" shakes, nature in as unadulterated a form as is possible. This consumption of nature is also a consumption of a kind of time. When chronic illness is conceptualized, it is often put into opposition to acute illness, but it may be useful to conceptualize the relationship between the event and the horizon. The event is discrete: it is the "flare up" and the experience of its treatment; the horizon recedes through treatment. Where the chronic and the acute both traffic in an experience of the event, both stand in opposition to the ungraspable horizon. That horizon is a therapeutic goal, and one that motivates personal actions, both dietary and medical, and might also be accepted as an attempt in this anthropogenic moment to conceptualize the long arc of human civilization and its relationship to the management of nature through a reincorporation of the human into nature, which depends on an inward and outward stewardship.

A question that lingers is that of disgust, or the "ick factor." Theories of disgust, dirt, and disorder all point to the eruptive potential of "matter out of place," or "flux," or the "abject." Surely, Peter's experimental use of excremental shakes and their depiction on video through Facebook is meant to elicit a visceral response in his audience, but this is tempered by his audience's understanding that what Peter is doing has a medical aim and is born of his desperation. The parallel efforts in the cookbooks discussed here are the authors' attempts to overcome the predispositions of the Standard American Diet, much like Kellogg and Davis before them. In their attempts to convince their readers of the essential merits of making broth with whole chicken carcasses and of eating cow tallow straight from the bone or of the need to eat copious amount of gelatin, they attempt to reconfigure American appetites to push the boundaries of a regime of disgust grounded in the Standard American Diet and unsettle disgust. In unsettling disgust, they also seek to dismember the human, making stewardship as a personal practice central to human interactions with self and other, and thereby implicitly making humans the caretakers of their food-providing environments and the colony within, immune from dependence on other humans who may be risky FMT donors, yet integrally tied to the environment and the curatives it provides.

## The Excremental Horizon

If pooineership and "pioneer science shit" rely on the shared understanding that the science and medicine of FMT is neutral, serving as a means to relatively effortlessly replace one microbial colony with another, discussions of race and ethnicity in relation to donors show how FMT seekers are shaping the practice of FMT through implicit and explicit conceptions of race and the permeability of bodies. Their understandings of FMT's potentials are positive and negative, but racist nonetheless. FMT seeker attitudes cannot and should not be dissociated from the medical and scientific conceptions of FMT as neutral; the dangers that physicians, scientists, and state agencies have associated with FMT are nebulous and based entirely on the content of the donor sample, not the procedure itself. It is precisely because FMT has been carefully constructed by advocates as a safe procedure, and the contents it conveys as the source of any danger, that these racist associations are able to adhere to the content of the donor sample and the donors who provide the excremental medicine. The dangers that FMT seekers and recipients focus on are racial anxieties and fears of kinship that the neutral conduit of FMT makes possible. Likeness, or similitude, becomes something that is transmissible through technological means, transferring colonies between individuals and potentially colonizing whole populations of sick individuals through the unwitting actions of careless physicians. The microbial colony emerges as a site of contestation precisely because it returns attention to concerns with race that science and politics have sought to bury in discourses of postracial societies and biologies. Race returns, again, not as a marker of phenotypic alterity, but as a vector of transformation from within to be guarded against, a return of the settler-colonial repressed.

Stewardship stands in opposition to the human-to-human interdependence that FMT implies. As a practice, FMT seeks to provide individuals with the ability to care for themselves in ways that reflect the environmental interdependence that all living creatures have, tied to their food sources and environmental exposures; the healthy steward is a curator of one's microbial colony through careful diet and, by extension, the environment that makes that diet possible. In the context of a consumerist society, this secondary aspect of stewardship is diffuse: it becomes possible through what people choose to buy, where they choose to buy it, and the supply chains that make particular goods consumable. Rather than the one-to-one negotiations that FMT donations require, stewardship as consumption allows for an imagined independence predicated on one's economic means. The result is that the microbial becomes something someone consumes, not as a relation, but as a standardized and normalizing product. The rise of probiotics as consumable goods is an outgrowth of precisely this, itself dependent on the microbial being made consumable and desirable. Yogurt is not Peter's feces shake, nor does it have quite the same effect, microbially. But it is microbial medicine nonetheless—simply the kind many Americans find palatable and accessible. And, as a consumable good aimed at maintaining one's health among many other consumer products, it offers Americans the opportunity to steward the colony within.

# 7 Planetary Health, Scalar Bodies, and the Impossible Turn to Microbial Medicine

HOW DOES THE INDIVIDUAL STEWARD THE PLANETARY? That question lies at the heart of planetary health, a medical-governmental-scholarly effort to connect changes in the environment with individual health and behavior. Foundationally, it builds on the Centers for Disease Control's OneHealth approach, the project to convey the interconnectedness of human health with nonhuman animal health, environmental sustainability, and the environmental conveyance of disease vectors, which sought to find ways to make people care about how their actions led to downstream health effects for humans, nonhumans, and environments. But planetary health scales up from there. Where OneHealth might seek to connect communities and actors in a relatively circumscribed context, planetary health seeks to describe the interdependence of all life on Earth. With this as its justification, planetary-health practitioners—which include a diverse array of scholars, policy makers, and activists—connect individual bodies and behaviors with dangers to the planet and well-being around the world. In this way, the individual becomes planetary, their body cast as an extension of the world. Choices like what one eats or how one travels or whether one chooses to have children are all cast as having an impact on the planet. On one level, it feels like the inevitable outcome of a century of American environmentalism; on another level, it is an intensification of American liberalism that individualizes responsibility for collective needs and depends on the motivational understanding that some people are doing the "right" thing while others are not. This, in turn, depends on the cultivation of a kind of disgust that finds its leverage not in kinds of people, nor kinds of substances, but kinds of practices. It is an abstract disgust that motivates the embodiment of scale: I am the body of the world, the world is an extension of my body. Such a conception of scale also motivates conceptualizing other people's bodies and the practices they engage in as threatening the planet and my body. Where earlier discourses about dieting and self-care targeted individual bodies for the abstract threats they engendered toward the public weal, now they threaten the Earth itself. What better justification could exist to regulate the bodies of others? In this way, planetary health is the apotheosis of American settler colonialism. It grounds the domination of bodies in scientific rationales and strives toward global homogeneity. That might be strong language for a project that seems benign, but its underlying logic is grounded in changing individual behaviors rather than confronting systemic reform to facilitate people living the lives they want to lead.

In 2013, the Rockefeller Foundation led an effort in the development of planetary health. As a rubric, it was intended to bring together experts in the social, medical, and geophysical sciences, with an eye toward forwarding interventions to improve the health of humans, nonhumans, and the Earth. Growing out of the emerging literature on the Anthropocene, particularly in the social sciences, planetary health has sought to show how impacts to the natural environment have downstream effects for human and nonhuman health. It has also attempted to show how a focus on the corporate and capitalist forces that compel everyday forms of consumption lead to feedback systems that compound environmental degradation and inequities in human health and disease. To date, as represented in the new journal *Lancet Planetary Health,* most contributions to planetary health focus on cohort studies of disease susceptibility, with a preponderance of studies on the effects of environmental pollutants on human populations.

The authors of the 2015 report by the Rockefeller Foundation–Lancet Commission on Planetary Health, *Safeguarding Human Health in the Anthropocene Epoch,* summarize a variety of now widely accepted threats to environmental stability that they argue have impacts on human health and well-being. Most of the environmental damages are associated with human "civilization" in the authors' reckoning, including rising global temperatures, increasing drought, ocean acidification, heat islands, and disruptions to food systems, which the authors argue are themselves too dependent on global trade and monocrops. These damages are exacerbated by the forces of overpopulation and carbon-based fuel consumption, and the resource extraction that is driven by these forces. They argue that human health has been enabled and sustained through a relationship with "nature" that was roughly constant up until the Anthropocene, when industrial production began to alter the atmosphere, water table, and food system, and led to a quickening of the process of overpopulation and resource depletion previously discussed at least as far back as Thomas Malthus.[1] "Development," by which the authors mean industrialization as the primary aim of social change over time, is both the aspirational state that communities seek and the motor driving environmental degradation and dangers to human health. As a set of assumptions, the authors of the Rockefeller–Lancet report echo arguments made by a host of other scholars and journalists focused on the Anthropocene, adding to the effects of environmental degradation the widespread risks to human health and well-being that move beyond those in close proximity to current developmental efforts, suggesting that global populations are increasingly at risk as a result of historic and contemporary pollution related to production and consumption. In this way, the authors of the report seek not to establish a new paradigm, but extend the current understanding of the Anthropocene to include detrimental effects to human health, and thereby motivate policy interventions that overcome political impasses in the present.

The authors of the Rockefeller–Lancet report posit that the challenge facing us as a global community is threefold: "imagination challenges," "research and information challenges," and "governance challenges."[2] Among the first, they suggest that "conceptual" and "empathy" failures are characterized by the inability to work beyond economistic metrics of well-being (e.g., gross domestic product [GDP]) and to be aware that other communities and individuals may be negatively affected by processes remote to them (e.g., communities displaced due to sea-level rise as a result of carbon-dioxide emissions they did not cause, as in the case of the Maldives). Barriers to knowledge, captured in "research and information challenges," include "an increasingly molecular approach to medicine, which ignores social and environmental context,"[3] a point that echoes—albeit with an inversion—the rise of microbial medicine. Finally, the failures of governments and other institutions to implement formal regulations represent "governance challenges" that might be confronted through "adaptive" and, more importantly, "transformational" strategies that not only adapt to current conditions, but anticipate continued changes in the environment and their potential downstream effects on human health. These three "challenges" are bound together through forms of structural racism that were codified in the context of colonialism and intensified through industrial and neoliberal capitalism.[4]

At the heart of the Rockefeller–Lancet report are a set of suggestions for how to address these threats to human and planetary health. Across the recommendations, the authors of the report seek to join macro level initiatives focusing on policy to lived experiences of everyday life, thereby changing both how governments act and how individuals and communities address their perceived needs. In so doing, they seek to create planetary health as a scalar object that joins everyday action with planetary effects, both for one's individual life and also for unseen others. Among their recommendations are: founding systems of ethics and values that protect future generations, address inequalities, and promote safe and just operating systems; building resilience among communities so as to weather catastrophic climate changes; monetizing nonmarket benefits that would incentivize individuals and communities to emphasize alternative forms of labor; moving beyond a "circular economy" of consumption-driven labor; moving the measurement of human progress and well-being away from economistic reductions to GDP and toward metrics that more clearly capture lived human experience; and imposing taxation and generating subsidies to support planetary health through economic incentives and disincentives.[5] What they seek to do, without naming it as such, is move away from the neoliberal culture of the North Atlantic, which has successfully spread through cultural and economic globalization, and replace it with a communitarian social structure that emphasizes collective effects of individual action. To effect this change, they seek to change the economic basis of contemporary governance and everyday life, moving away from neoliberal incentives for self-promotion and toward collective protection and intergenerational care.

In making this argument, the authors rely on a set of concepts that work across scale, from individuals' lives to social formations. "Human civilization," "resilience," "adaptation," "governance," and "development" serve this function. As a set of imbricated concepts, they serve to reify civilization as an inevitable outcome of the developmental impulses that capitalism in the North Atlantic set into motion in the context of mercantilism and intensified through extractive colonial and industrial practices.[6] In this way, they imply both that human motivations are exquisitely realized in liberal and neoliberal capitalism and that human desires can be changed through an alteration to the economic system that would produce new forms of social value. The underside of this reification of human nature in the forces of capitalism are twofold: first, without a clear conception of the plasticity of "human nature" and how it can be fundamentally changed through social drivers, like the economy, it implies that human societies will revert back to some form of extractive capitalism over time;[7] secondly, it inadvertently suggests that capacities like "resilience" and "adaptation" are the inborn qualities of particular individuals and communities, with some individuals "naturally" being able to maintain themselves or adapt to outside forces while others are not able.[8] In both cases, how capitalism and colonialism have shaped "human nature" and capacities like "resilience" and "adaptation" remains uninterrogated; yet, because of the ways that they see global communities as interconnected, they seek to provide a way to overcome any conceptual bias that disfavors individuals and communities by fundamentally changing the systemic forces that continue to disadvantage some communities and compound forms of neocolonial racism and inequity.

Ultimately, they argue that the turn to planetary health requires the development of new coalitions of experts who can successfully frame the issues facing global populations in ways that will compel action on the part of governments to make significant, transformative changes to mitigate climate change and its social effects.

> Planetary health will have to build novel coalitions to achieve meaningful and lasting change. Communities struggling to preserve their environments and livelihoods need scientists and health leaders to engage on their issues, document their suffering, and work with them to create social change. The scientific and health communities, in turn, will be much more successful in influencing decision makers who are

feeling pressure for change from their constituents than they would without the support of civil society.[9]

In evoking "suffering," they appeal to the liberal sensibility that human suffering is a universal and knowable, if not entirely objective, feature of human life, and that its documentation is unproblematic.[10] Attention to "suffering" depends on a shared conception of human life and its value as motivating attention to human rights that would secure individuals and communities against the structural forms of violence that produce and maintain the precarity that entails widespread human suffering.[11] The challenge is that the presumed liberal moral of valuing human life is not as widely shared as needed to make systemic changes, and that, in many cases, this liberal value depends on its own violences that grow out of colonial and postcolonial race relations.[12]

The analysis in the report exists at the macro level of markets, governments, and the other largely public institutions that structure everyday life. When providing case reports from rural South Africa,[13] the Ebola outbreak in the Democratic Republic of Congo,[14] the health and economic effects of environmental degradation in Pakistan (1996), ecological restoration as an economic driver in the Loess Plateau in China (2004), and the damage to communities as a result of Hurricane Katrina in Louisiana (2009), the authors situate their analysis at the level of policy as a response to environmental forces. The most obvious omissions in the choice of case studies—all of which focus on racialized populations, most of them outside of the North Atlantic—are the white communities who, through their labor and consumption, have driven ecological degradation since industrialization. This is clear in the white rural communities who are invested in the status quo as much as the suburban and urban communities that depend on the contemporary capitalist global order to support their ways of life.[15] What they also tend to ignore—and this may be an artifact of the authors' approach, which seeks to array the macro-level strictures and influences that compel further environmental damage and threaten human health—is the level of individual everyday life that captures how people think and act, and under what conditions individuals and communities decide to enact significant changes. It's in this context that the planetary-health diet seeks to individualize the moral burden of planetary health, and here where the history of American settler-colonialism comes into renewed contact with a compulsion to steward the globe and its people through neocolonial practice.

In 2019, a report was published by the EAT-Lancet Commission entitled *Food in the Anthropocene: the EAT-Lancet Commission on health diets from sustainable food systems.*[16] The commission was composed of scholars and practitioners from around the world and drew from a broad interdisciplinary collection of perspectives, with leadership in epidemiology. The aim of the commission, as indexed by the title of the report, was to prepare a guide for the development of healthy diets around the world while abiding by the growing evidence provided by the environmental sciences about sustainable agricultural practices. On the surface, it's an admirable project: a global collection of thought-leaders brought together to integrate a variety of scientific perspectives in pursuit of creating the conditions for a healthy, sustainable human population. And where earlier generations might have balked at the problem of a growing population and suggested straightforwardly eugenic policies, the EAT-Lancet Commission does no such thing. Instead, they offer a seemingly value-neutral set of recommendations that are, nonetheless, suffused with values.

The executive summary and a podcast that were prepared by the EAT-Lancet Commission provide the public face of the effort. The official report was aimed at a more scholarly audience, and its language is measured to reach that audience; but the language of the executive summary imagines another audience entirely, and engages in forms of rhetorical work that seek to make the stakes of adopting the EAT-Lancet Commission's recommendations personal. These stakes are about both the diets and the everyday practices of individuals and the conditions of the globe, specifically the Earth's ability to sustain human and nonhuman life. In this way, it creates a parallelism between the lived experience of individuals and the policy contexts that ground the conditions of those everyday experiences: it seeks to somaticize the global and to make the future of the planet a personal one that the individual is charged with stewarding through relationships with food, nonhuman others, and the environment.

In order to make the global personal, the EAT-Lancet Commission casts the risks faced by individuals as analogous to the risks faced by the planet. This is accomplished by creating a connection between "unhealthy diets" for individuals and their impacts on the planet through deforestation and pollution. "Unhealthy diets now pose a greater risk to morbidity and mortality than unsafe sex, alcohol, drug and tobacco use combined. . . . The boundaries of the safe [environmental] operating space are placed at the lower end of the scientific uncertainty range, establishing a 'safe space' which, if transgressed, would push humanity into an uncertainty zone of rising risks."[17] Health serves as a "boundary" for the individual, and eating unhealthy diets risks rupturing that boundary and placing individuals in situations of disease. In making these claims, the authors minimize how rates of tobacco and alcohol use have decreased over the last century and treatments for diseases associated with sexually transmitted infections, drug use, and other "lifestyle" conditions have improved in efficacy. The relative impacts of diet are harder to discern, since it is difficult to isolate diet as a single variable, but in the wake of an ongoing "war on obesity," diet serves as a means to do the rhetorical work of convincing people to change their behaviors. Later, the authors of the executive summary write: "Dietary changes from current diets toward healthy diets are likely to result in major health benefits. This includes preventing approximately 11 million deaths per year, which represents between 19% and 24% of total deaths among adults."[18] Here, "diet" serves as a fulcrum to connect individual practice to the global situation of the Anthropocene, and mortality rates scale between the individual and the planetary; individual behaviors reflect the conditions of possibility (what one can eat and what one wants to eat) and influence the conditions of the future, both for the individual and the world. Might one eater's decisions put them into or outside of that "preventable" 11 million deaths per year? Might careful dietary choices reduce the risk of my neighbor's death? The EAT-Lancet Commission is banking on its audience accepting that premise to the degree that alterations in their diet feel like an appropriate response.

On the *Let's Rethink Food* podcast, produced in support of the EAT-Lancet report as a means to publicize its finding, one of its leaders, Johan Rockström makes the following statement, which puts a fine point on connecting the personal and the planetary through "health":

We can now scientifically create a compelling joint story where many of the health benefits of food also are planetary benefits of food. And I would even argue that [unintelligible] from a sustainability perspective that that health argument is a vector to succeed on sustainability. Because quite frankly it's not easy to communicate sustainability always. You know, why should I save the planet? But on the health—given you actually can reach the hearts of individuals directly. It's very personal. It comes down to, to me as an individual. Do I or don't I want to have a healthy life?

Rockström takes the abstractions of the executive summary and puts them into directly personal terms: "Do I or don't I want to have a healthy life?" If the question were that simple, the answer would be an unequivocal "yes" for many, but the question becomes one of means, and this is where the problem of the planetary-health diet resides and what I find so troubling, bordering on disgusting.

Walter Willett, the lead author on the EAT-Lancet Commission report, describes the diet as "flexitarian." Largely vegetarian in its assumptions, the planetary-health diet consists of vegetable-based proteins with the possibility of very small amounts of meat proteins and dairy. These recommendations are based on the awareness that the environmental effects of livestock farming are a primary driver in environmental degradation, leading to localized forms of toxic pollution around livestock farms and planetary climate changes as a result of deforestation in favor of land appropriated for raising cows for global markets. The authors of the executive summary describe the diet as additionally flexible in relation to "local interpretations."

> Although the planetary health diet, which is based on health considerations, is consistent with many traditional eating patterns, it does not imply that the global population should eat exactly the same food, nor does it prescribe an exact diet. . . . Local interpretations and adaptation of the universally-acceptable planetary health diet is necessary and should reflect the culture, geography and demography of the population and individuals.[19]

The diet is intended to be open to "local interpretations," allowing for people and communities to inflect it with dietary practices that reflect the demands of the diet while also aligning with individual and local forms of taste. When the authors of the diet write that "opponents will warn of unintended consequences or argue that the case for action is premature or should be left to existing dynamics,"[20] they expose their ignorance about what's actually at stake in adopting a diet like the one they propose for many people.

Colonialism often comes with changes to local foodways, imposing the diets of imperial centers on people in their colonies. This can mean the replacement of everyday crops with those preferred by imperial elites; it can also involve the scientific displacement of foodways in support of making the diets of the colonized appear more like the diets preferred by those in power. This can lead to the replacement of sustainable foodways that have developed over generations and are in accord with seasonal and regional flora and fauna with foodways that depend on industrial production and global distribution networks. This has been the case for Indigenous communities throughout North America, nowhere more apparent that among Inuit communities, where reliance on seal meat has been a site of recurrent intervention, both during explicitly colonial periods and as interventions into postcolonial lifeways.[21] Drawing as they do on local resources, traditional Inuit diets are relatively light on fruits and vegetables, instead depending on vitamins and minerals found in fresh meat. The sustainability and healthiness of a traditional Inuit diet has decreased because of disruptions to everyday life, from the structure of labor and housing to the demands of capitalist markets. The planetary-health diet seeks to rectify a problem that earlier forms of colonialism created. It does so by imposing a form of colonialism without content: a form of regulation that conceals itself through its apparent neutrality. "Flexitarianism" hides within it the displacement of foodways like that of Inuit communities. Who could object to a diet that appears so reasonable, so connected to individual and planetary health?

Is it too much to say that my affective response to the planetary-health diet is one of disgust? I write this as a "flexitarian," someone who has been largely vegetarian for most of my life, with a sparing amount of seafood eaten while traveling or on holidays. In the same episode of *Let's Rethink Food* mentioned above, Willet refers to the planetary-health diet as aligned with the Mediterranean diet, a "blue zone" fantasy that claims that the traditional diet of people in the Greek islands promotes longevity and healthiness. Like the merits of a great-books education based entirely in the literary and philosophical traditions of Europe and North America, an appeal to one "flexitarian" tradition over others—for example, instead of the vegetarianism of Buddhist and Hindu communities—is a rationalization grounded in the appeal of an archaic whiteness. An appeal to a "traditional" diet without attention to how colonialism has disrupted and displaced other lifeways erodes the legitimacy of other practices that might have been sustainable and healthy before colonial impositions. My disgust is rooted in my implication. Inasmuch as the politics of the movement for planetary health and the structure of its diet might be my own, their radical dehistoricization and insensitivity to local lifeways make it an imperial project quite different from my diet and political commitments. Theirs is a form of whiteness that seeks to conceal itself through the canny composition of a multinational committee and a diet that is largely contentless; in seeking to skirt objection, they have composed a meal that is textureless and bland. A truly planetary diet would do something different: reimagine sustainability through local lifeways that unsettle the lingering power of imperialism and the dietary displacements it engendered, while also critiquing the dominant ways of conceptualizing health and well-being based in North Atlantic body ideals that have been guided by deeply somaticized experiences of disgust grounded in settler-colonial encounters and the American development of whiteness. That project is necessarily multiscalar and multispecies.

The cultivation of disgust helps to make the world small. Scale has been approached from a variety of directions, from the discursive construction of registers, to the molding of a child's sensibilities to reflect a social order, to the enactment of scientific expertise and power. In each of these cases, scale is something that is lived, as people and communities encounter frictions based on the mismatches between conceptual scales and everyday experience. In order for scale to work through embodiment, affective states need to be cultivated to ensure that scale operates in the ways that those in power seek to make tangible. Disgust does this work, creating the conditions for ideas about what can pass into and through a body and what a body can be in contact with, thereby connecting it to the environment it is part of through the food one eats and the medicine one consumes. A tightly wound sense of disgust facilitates the consumption of certain things over others, interactions with some substances and not others, and relationships between some people and not others. That is how and why disgust is so central to the colonial project,[22] both in its imperial phase and in contemporary biomedicine, wherein some substances are safe (e.g., pharmaceuticals) and others are not (e.g., fecal microbial transplant [FMT]).

In the context of American capitalist, consumerist society, these concerns with scale are laminated on consumable goods and how they circulate. When goods circulate outside of markets, unlike prescribed medicines, which are multiply regulated by health care providers, pharmacists, and insurance providers in the United States, then a sense of disgust can intervene to ensure that some things are not consumed or are consumed in ways that are circumscribed by circumstances that only particular individuals and communities have access to. Such is the case with FMTs, which only some Americans have formal access to through proximity to health-care providers skilled in its delivery; and for those who lack such access, the "ick factor" intervenes to ensure that self-administered microbial transplants are undesirable—except in cases of desperation. Desperation sunders scale.

But desperation is a product of its social context as well, and the kinds of diseases individuals are exposed to and the medicines they have available to them make certain experiences of desperation possible, and lay the grounds for the alleviation of that desperation. In the case of the administration of FMTs, it is both biomedicine's dependence on antibiotics that create the conditions for microbial dysbiosis and the conditions in which microbial infusions might cure them. The challenge that individuals face is not the procedure, but the dismantling of their disgust. That disgust and its dismembering necessarily occurs in the context of settler-colonial relations and the legacies and lived realities of American racism and ableism, which influence what bodies people are willing to be exposed to and how they manage those exposures. In this way, disgust works and reworks the embodiment of scale through the biology of everyday life, those intercalated experiences of physiological capacities, social norms, and cultural expectations that create the conditions of possibility and guide what is consumed, how it is consumed, and what relations that consumption produces.

"Embodiment" is insufficient to conceptualize how the biology of everyday life is lived in the context of a more-than-human ecosystem in which the human body is merely one element. Instead, "somatization" captures how individual human bodies are composed of a diverse array of microbial and other elements that shape and are shaped by human life. Disgust, then, is not simply an individually enculturated response, but a systemic reaction of which a seemingly personal action is a metonym of cultural expectations, institutionalized social organization, and physiological capacities. Disgust is also generative and generating, helping to recompose the biology of everyday life as an expression of the possible, at the individual level and across scale. Disgust is protective of individual lifeways, society as a whole, and the ecosystems through which human life is composed. Yet, it is often deployed in ways that harm and limit, that traffic in racism, speciesism, and human exceptionality, all of which are steeped in whiteness and its forms of exclusion. Understanding this is a step toward accepting the rooting of disgust in self-preservation and moral orders not as politically neutral and grounded in a universal human nature, but as inculcated tools of those in power who seek to preserve exclusionary social orders and continue colonialism by other means.

In the days that followed my drinking pickle juice, I would swear that I had an effervescent feeling in my gut. It felt as if there was a chorus of activity, as if my gut had been infused with a wave of activity unlike its usual staid complacency. I felt oddly responsible to keep the party going and made sure to eat yogurt and kimchi regularly in the days that followed; I also tapped into my partner's kombucha in the refrigerator. But after a few days, whatever had originally been happening as a result of the initial lacto-fermented infusion, real or imagined, seemed to die down and I felt a return to my normal gut activity. For the brief moment in which things seemed to be different, I wondered whether all of the gut-related speculation I had been consuming, all of the diet books and websites, were really onto something, and whether this was the kind of stewardship that they encouraged people toward. But the reality of it, for me at least, was that to maintain the feeling of something different in the gut meant kinds of food consumption at levels that I was unprepared for committing to as part of my everyday diet. Had I had an ongoing gastrointestinal concern, I may have made other choices, but given my relatively normal (I think?) digestion, it seemed like too much work for an uncertain effect. That may paint me as unsympathetic to my gut and its health; maybe it could be much better and what the pickle juice infusion had done was provide me with a momentary experience of that other possibility. Given my history and willingness to experiment, it also felt like I could return to the experiment as needed. The microbial remains a possibility, even if it is not something I have entirely embraced.

In flirting with the microbial in my consumption of that jar of pickle juice, I may have also been flirting with unsettling disgust. If only for a moment, that moment before a first sip, I had to confront an emergent disgust, something a little wild. This was a domesticated disgust and something that I confronted in my home related to things we already consumed; it was just on the edge of everyday life and not unsettling in a profound way. Even the kinds of disgust that I have confronted as a parent, from cleaning a child's poopy butt to finding myself finishing a half-eaten piece of food left by a child, are always momentary and become, respectively, elements of everyday life ("poop is just poop!" I tell my children) or the basis for better decision-making (I don't need to finish someone else's uneaten food). Disgust may be protective at times, but it is equally important to work through it to make the everyday possible; where disgust bleeds into the abject, though, sets a boundary on the possibilities of the everyday, the abject serving as the limit of the possible. Where the abject and desperation meet, we might find the real potentials of unsettling disgust.

Unsettling disgust is necessarily a project focused on what we put into our bodies and the interaction between bodies, both as persons encountering other persons and persons encountering nonhumans. The histories of colonialism and liberalism have recurrently placed certain kinds of people outside of personhood and nonhumans outside of humane regard. In both cases, disgust has been central to the self-regulation of individuals who might come into contact with these forms of difference, and grooming that disgust as a "civilized" reaction was necessary to uphold the white supremacist powers of dominant institutions and people. Something as mundane as different foodways could elicit disgust; and discourses of miscegenation often played on ideas about abject bodies and sexual temperaments. We may find ourselves far removed from such attitudes in our everyday lives, but the question might be: how much of everyday life has been constructed to protect ourselves from an experience of disgust? I imagine that for many people, disgust exists at the edges of the everyday. What is your pickle jar and how might you drink from it? And, from there, where else might you encounter disgust in more profound and unsettling ways, from which to articulate new sensibilities of the possible?

If much of this history of food and disgust, medicine and magic, racism and ableism, and excrement and dirt is also a story about biomedicine's unsympathetic relations to the microbial, then embracing disgust may also be an embrace of a sympathetic medicine, a form of medicine that makes new forms of living possible. If unsympathetic medicine has been characterized by its dependence on cure and the cessation or elimination of disease, a sympathetic medicine might instead embrace the possibility of likeness, of making one body like another through the sharing of capacities or complementary qualities of another body. The rejection of difference in racist attitudes toward FMT donors, as recounted in chapter 6, might be usefully inverted so as to facilitate the use of unconventional— and sometimes maligned—medicines. These medicines might not be excremental in the strict sense, although FMT may be part of an expanded materia medica, but they might develop out of recent research on nonhuman therapeutics, from the consumption of helminths and other parasites to the experimental use of phages to combat microbial infections.[23] While we are usefully wary of some kinds of exposures, what exposures of the possible is an unsympathetic medicine needlessly protecting us from? The challenge may be divorcing such sympathetic medicines from overarching and overdetermining ideas about nature and a return to primordial forms of health that exclude as much as they make possible. A truly sympathetic medicine necessitates the embrace of a symmetrical relationship between bodies and forms of life in ways that dismember the human as an individualized and independent object and instead situate it as one body among many in an ecosystem of interdependencies. Recomposing the human as a site of relations rather than a discrete object sets the conditions for reconceptualizing the possible, both in terms of human well-being and in terms of environmental stewardship, based immediately in the care of the self but extending to our local and planetary environments.

The promise of microbial medicine is that it undoes the unsympathetic affects that suffuse medicine and its practice as Americans have inherited it. Planetary health, dietary activism, and William Beaumont's experiments on Alexis St. Martin are all moments in this history, as are the practices endorsed by John Harvey Kellogg and contributors to the natural-foods movements of the twentieth century. But attention to the microbial recomposes the world in another way that, instead of situating the body as an isolated and endangered object threatened by elements from without, accepts that the body is a porous, molecular and microbial landscape that exists in continuous relations with microbial agents in its local environments. These environments are surely impacted by global processes, but the homogenous approach endorsed by efforts like "planetary health" erodes local foodways and practices of sustainability with a carefully constructed neutrality that obscures its whiteness and colonial influences. A more sympathetic practice (one that lies in my experiments with pickle juice and the efforts of FMT providers and seekers) attends to how our bodies are made through interpersonal, microbial, and environmental relations and seeks to find sustainable ways to make worldly well-being desirable and attainable. Unsettling disgust is one means toward this end, but is only just the beginning.

But as an ending, I find this beginning unsatisfactory. It doesn't sit well with me. My dalliance with pickle juice individualizes something that should be collective: accepting the body as landscape implicates the participation of every other person, human and nonhuman, who inhabits that landscape. That it is left to me alone as an experimentalist ratifies the experiences of desperation that FMT seekers have that allows them to move through their feelings of disgust and toward some form of remedy; we are left to fend for ourselves for the benefit of each of us as individuals, but potentially with benefits to our shared environment as a byproduct of those actions. Planetary health offers another model—potentially. In its current mode, planetary health has too often sought to individualize responsibility, as in the case of the planetary-health diet, which extends a century or more of right-living that has resonated throughout American approaches to health and well-being. When planetary health doesn't individualize responsibility, it falls back on neocolonial models of imposing ways of living on communities and individuals with little attention to local ways of knowing and practice. In so doing, planetary health can motivate old conceptions of disgust as targeting people's ways of life, if not people themselves; it's the same project, same narratives, cloaked in another neocolonial effort to impose a form of order on disorder, sameness on difference. Unsettling disgust might provide another way to imagine and bring into being a collective future aimed at the care of humans and nonhumans and the environments they inhabit. As an ongoing and always-unresolved project, unsettling disgust demands encountering the new—or encountering the old with the capacity to change one's reactions to it. Disgust may be a barrier, but it isn't an impenetrable one. Instead, it is porous and allows for change, for the passage through disgust into another affective state. Identifying where disgust resides, both individually and collectively, and finding means through that disgust is the promise that its unsettling provides. In a straightforward way, the FDA could provide widespread approval, support, and access to FMTs, which would signify the acceptance of the procedure governmentally. This might lower the threshold of disgust for many patients and their families; it might also lower this threshold and raise the acceptance of health-care providers. This imposition of acceptance could also motivate approaches to planetary health, where, rather than proscriptive models emanating from the North Atlantic and the affluent, partnerships with local communities could develop sustainable and sensitive approaches to communal life. How we get to this collaborative future is by overcoming our barriers to living together, with our human and nonhuman cohabitants. There are no easy routes, only the constant project of unsettling ourselves, individually and collectively, toward a common future.

# Acknowledgments

This project languished on the back burner of my work stove for nearly a decade, and over that time developed in unpredictable ways until it reached a point where I almost never wrote this book: it could be so many things that deciding what one thing it needed to be became remote to me. But then the Covid-19 pandemic happened and what I thought my next project was going to be became impossible, and I took the time to survey what was already cooking to determine whether any of it could become something. I distinctly remember driving my children back from a walk in the gorges of Ithaca and working through the possibilities of what could go into this book, coming to accept that it couldn't be everything but just had to be one thing.

Around the same time, a conversation with my editor, Jason Weidemann, resulted in some subtle peer pressure. Jason's insistence that "people are ready" for this book was heartening, even if I wasn't entirely convinced. But I needed some kind of project to focus on to mitigate my pandemic anxieties, and this became that project. I asked my partner, Katherine Martineau, to join Jason in peer-pressuring me to work on the book, which she was game for, and I started to make plodding progress on putting everything together. My deepest thanks goes to them both for their encouragement and their abilities to anticipate what this project could become, even when I couldn't.

What made the book more possible was receiving a fellowship from the Institute for Advanced Study at Tampere University in Finland. Despite logistical difficulties—exacerbated by the pandemic—it provided two years of concentrated writing and research time. It also provided opportunities to be in dialogue with colleagues throughout Europe, which refined my commitments to being an Americanist and writing scholarship as a form of critique. My deepest gratitude goes to Juha Teperi and Marjukka Virkajärvi for all of their work on making my family's time in Finland possible; my thanks for jovial, expatriate companionship go to Tom Apperley, who helped us manage our way through a big move. My thanks to Laura Huttunen, who demonstrated what a warm and supportive place an anthropology department can be, and to Anna Rastas for encouraging me to work through my assumptions about race and racialization and the kinds of things that make their American iterations particular. Similarly, my thanks to Pekka Louhiala, who, over several cups of coffee, encouraged me to work through some of my assumptions about the history of American medicine and how it has shaped practices and bodies. And my thanks to two very different historians, Fa-ti Fan and Ville Kivimäki, for their encouragements to attend to the comparative complexities of telling American stories.

Henni Alava and her family—Mikko, Eemil, Wilho, and Hilja—made our time in Finland exceptionally fun and warm, and I will always appreciate how they made us feel at home in a foreign place. I will also always appreciate the food tourism that Henni facilitated, and her commitment to expanding our culinary horizons. My extra thanks to Henni for providing me with opportunities to talk through elements of this book even when she didn't know that's what we were doing, and likely neither did I.

Being in Finland also brought me into conversation with Salla Sariola and the creative and curious group of scholars associated with the Centre for the Social Study of Microbes. My very special thanks to Salla for all of her enthusiasm and support and to everyone who participated in a workshop focusing on the completion of this book. Maya Hey deserves a special thanks for time spent talking through the past and future of food studies, which I deeply appreciated.

Maria Pirogovskaya and Tamar Novick worked diligently to bring me to the Max Planck Institute for the History of Science and hosted a workshop about the book manuscript that pushed me through the final revisions. My thanks to them and to everyone who participated in the workshop—it made the last weeks of working on the project decidedly more possible. Special thanks to Gretchen Bakke and Lauren Cubellis for going out of their respective ways to join that conversation and to prompt me to work through my assumptions about parenting and its American histories.

The first time I presented anything related to this work was at an American Anthropological Association meeting on a panel with Karen-Sue Taussig, Seth Messinger, and Anna Zogas. I kept their early encouragement through the years and appreciated all of the counsel Seth and Karen-Sue provided in the interim. Around the same time, Will Garriott and Kevin Karpiak encouraged me to work through the relationship between policing and medicine, which resulted in a strange chapter in an edited volume that mutated into something else herein. My thanks to them—and to everyone who served as peer reviewers and editors, including Lance Gravlee, Vincanne Adams, Dana-ain Davis, and Sameena Mulla, of the bits and pieces that were eventually woven together into this book.

My thanks extend to the hosts and audiences of talks that I have given over the years that have drawn from this book and its many parts. Those include Rice University; University of Wisconsin, Madison; University of Copenhagen; University of Glasgow; Durham University; and the annual American Anthropological Association and Society for the Social Study of Science meetings. My thanks to Wendy Wall for her support at Binghamton University's Institute for Advanced Studies in the Humanities.

During the pandemic, access to archives was complicated. I deeply appreciate the support provided to me by archivists at the General Mills' archives in Minneapolis and the Andover Center for History & Culture, without whom the foray into the history of American yogurt would have been impossible.

So many friends have been roped into working through this project with me, whether they knew it at the time or not. Thanks, especially, to Charles Briggs, Celina Callahan-Kapoor, Beth Cohen, Stefan Ecks, Denielle Elliott, Michele Friedner, Nick Kawa, Paul Manning, John Marlovits, Eli Nadeau, Katy Overstreet, Eugene Raikhel, and Laura Stark for serving as spurs to work through particularly thorny issues.

The staff at the University of Minnesota Press are consistently excellent, and writing books is made possible knowing that they receive the kind of care they do from the editorial, design, production, and marketing teams there. My thanks to everyone, but especially to Zenyse Miller and Jason Weidemann, who do the dirty work of getting me through the process. My thanks, also, to the two peer reviewers who helped hone the book into its final form.

As always, my deepest gratitude goes to my family. To say that this book wouldn't exist without the lessons that my children have taught me is an understatement of the grossest sort. Felix and Iggy, in their turn and consistently, encourage me to grapple with the histories and presents of being a parent and the need to address the diverse needs, desires, and capacities of other people. It has been a constant education and its benefits are ongoing. Their willingness to approach the body and social mores playfully is always inspiring, and even though we rarely play games of "Rude or Not Rude" these days, their lessons stick with me. Our dog Starling was a constant companion through the writing of the book, and although she is officially retired, I appreciate all of the subtle emotional support she provided. My mother welcomed Starling into her house to facilitate our move to Finland, which was an enormous relief; it made everything else possible. My thanks to her for that and for all of the encouragement over the years. Similarly, my parents-in-law, Steve and Deb, helped make our transition to Finland possible, and I will always be appreciative of all they do to support us—and their curiosity and encouragement. And, finally, to my partner Katherine, I owe all the gratitude that remains. Thank you.

# Notes

## Preface

1. Faith Rohlke and Neil Stollman, "Fecal Microbiota Transplantation in Relapsing Clostridium Difficile Infection," *Therapeutic Advances in Gastroenterology* 5, no. 6 (2012): 403–20.

2. Jamie Lorimer, "Why Liberals Love the Microbiome," *Medical Anthropology Quarterly* (blog), 2017, medanthroquarterly.org/forums/forumreview/why-liberals-love-the-microbiome/.

3. Michael J. Montoya, *Making the Mexican Diabetic: Race, Science, and the Genetics of Inequality* (Berkeley: University of California Press, 2011); Deepa Reddy, "Good Gifts for the Common Good: Blood and Bioethics in the Market of Genetic Research," *Cultural Anthropology* 22, no. 3 (2007): 429–72; Karen-Sue Taussig, *Ordinary Genomes: Normalizing the Future through Genetic Research and Practice* (Durham, N.C.: Duke University Press, 2009).

4. Amber Benezra, Joseph DeStefano, and Jeffrey Gordon, "Anthropology of Microbes," *Proceedings of the National Academy of Sciences of the United States of America* 109, no. 17 (2012): 6378–81; Jamie Lorimer, "Gut Buddies: Multispecies Studies and the Microbiome," *Environmental Humanities* 8, no. 1 (2016): 57–76.

5. Warwick Anderson, *Colonial Pathologies: American Tropical Medicine, Race, and Hygiene in the Philippines* (Durham, N.C.: Duke University Press, 2006); James H. Jones, *Bad Blood: The Tuskegee Syphilis Experiment* (New York: Free Press, 1993); Adriana Petryna, *When Experiments Travel: Clinical Trials and the Global Search for Human Subjects* (Princeton, N.J.: Princeton University Press, 2009).

6. George Lakoff and Mark Johnson, *Metaphors We Live By* (Chicago: University of Chicago Press, 2003).

7. Rebecca Lester, *Famished: Eating Disorders and Failed Care in America* (Berkeley: University of California Press, 2019).

8. Bruno Latour, *The Pasteurization of France,* trans. Alan Sheridan (Cambridge, Mass.: Harvard University Press, 1988); Heather Paxson, *The Life of Cheese: Crafting Food and Value in America* (Berkeley: University of California Press, 2012).

## Introduction

1. Pierre Bourdieu, *Distinction: A Social Critique of the Judgement of Taste* (1984; repr. Cambridge, Mass.: Harvard University Press, 2000).

2. Drew Leder, *The Absent Body* (Chicago: University of Chicago Press, 1990).

3. Shigehisa Kuriyama, *The Expressiveness of the Body and the Divergence of Greek and Chinese Medicine* (New York: Zone, 1999).

4. David Armstrong, *A New History of Identity: A Sociology of Medical Knowledge* (New York: Palgrave, 2002); Dorothy Porter, *Health, Civilization and the State: A History of Public Health from Ancient to Modern Times* (New York: Routledge, 1999).

5. George Rosen, *A History of Public Health* (Baltimore: Johns Hopkins University Press, 1993); Charles Rosenberg, *Cholera Years: The United States in 1832, 1849, and 1866* (Chicago: University of Chicago Press, 1987).

6. Jacques Donzelot, *The Policing of Families,* trans. Robert Hurley (Baltimore, Md.: John Hopkins University Press, 1997); Michel Foucault, *The Birth of the Clinic: An Archaeology of Medical Perception,* trans. A. M. Sheridan Smith (New York: Vintage, 1994).

7. Dorothy Roberts, *Fatal Invention: How Science, Politics, and Big Business Re-Create Race in the Twenty-First Century* (New York: The New Press, 2011).

8. Kathleen Stewart, *Ordinary Affects* (Durham, N.C.: Duke University Press, 2007).

9. Norman Gevitz, ed., *Other Healers: Unorthodox Medicine in America* (Baltimore, Md.: Johns Hopkins University Press, 1988); Roy Porter, *The Greatest Benefit to Mankind: A Medical History of Humanity* (New York: Norton, 1999).

10. For a survey of categorical distinctions between "disease," "illness," and "sickness," consult Nancy Scheper-Hughes and Margaret Lock, "The Mindful Body: A Prolegomenon to Future Work in Medical Anthropology," *Medical Anthropology Quarterly* 1, no. 1 (1987): 6–41; Allan Young, "The Anthropologies of Illness and Sickness," *Annual Review of Anthropology* 11 (1982): 257–85.

11. James C. Whorton, *Nature Cures: The History of Alternative Medicine in America* (Oxford: Oxford University Press, 2002).

12. Paul Starr, *The Social Transformation of American Medicine* (New York: Basic, 1982).

13. Warwick Anderson, "Where Is the Postcolonial History of Medicine?," *Bulletin of the History of Medicine* 72, no. 3 (1998): 522–30; David Arnold, ed., *Imperial Medicine and Indigenous Societies* (Manchester: Manchester University Press, 1988); Shula Marks, "What Is Colonial about Colonial Medicine? And What Has Happened to Imperialism and Health?," *Social History of Medicine* 10, no. 2 (1997): 205–19.

14. Annette Kolodny, *The Lay of the Land: Metaphor as Experience and His-*

*tory in American Life and Letters* (Chapel Hill: University of North Carolina Press, 1984); Linda Nash, *Inescapable Ecologies: A History of Environment, Disease and Knowledge* (Berkeley: University of California Press, 2006); Henry Nash Smith, *Virgin Land: The American West as Symbol and Myth* (Cambridge, Mass.: Harvard University Press, 1978).

15. Lennard Davis, *Enforcing Normalcy: Disability, Deafness, and the Body* (New York: Verso, 1995); Rosemarie Garland Thomson, *Extraordinary Bodies: Figuring Physical Disability in American Culture and Literature* (New York: Columbia University Press, 1996); Sander L. Gilman, *Disease and Representation: Images of Illness from Madness to AIDS* (Ithaca, N.Y.: Cornell University Press, 1988).

16. Stephen Jay Gould, *The Mismeasure of Man* (New York: Norton, 1996); Oliver Rollins, *Conviction: The Making and Unmaking of the Violent Brain* (Palo Alto, Calif.: Stanford University Press, 2021).

17. James Doucet-Battle, "Sweet Salvation: One Black Church, Diabetes Outreach, and Trust," *Transforming Anthropology* 24, no. 2 (2016): 125–35; Don Kulick and Anne Meneley, eds., *Fat: The Anthropology of an Obsession* (New York: Penguin, 2005); Peter N. Stearns, *Fat History: Bodies and Beauty in the Modern West* (New York: New York University Press, 2002); Matthew Wolf-Meyer and Celina Callahan-Kapoor, "Chronic Subjunctivity, Or, How Physicians Use Diabetes and Insomnia to Manage Futures in the U.S.," *Medical Anthropology* 36, no. 2 (2017): 83–95.

18. Ashanté Reese, *Black Food Geographies: Race, Self-Reliance, and Food Access in Washington, D.C.* (Chapel Hill: University of North Carolina Press, 2019).

19. Matthew Wolf-Meyer, "Biomedicine, the Whiteness of Sleep and the Wages of Spatiotemporal Normativity," *American Ethnologist* 42, no. 3 (2015): 446–58.

20. Kalman Applbaum and Michael Oldani, "Towards an Era of Bureaucratically Controlled Medical Compliance?," *Anthropology & Medicine* 17, no. 2 (2010): 113–27.

21. Aurel Kolnai et al., *On Disgust* (Chicago: Open Court, 2004); Winfried Menninghaus, *Disgust: The Theory and History of a Strong Sensation,* Intersections (Albany: State University of New York Press, 2003); William Ian Miller, *The Anatomy of Disgust* (Cambridge, Mass.: Harvard University Press, 1997); Susan B. Miller, *Disgust: The Gatekeeper Emotion* (Hillsdale, N.J.: Analytic, 2004); Martha Craven Nussbaum, *Hiding from Humanity: Disgust, Shame, and the Law* (Princeton, N.J.: Princeton University Press, 2006); Parama Roy, *Alimentary Tracts: Appetites, Aversions, and the Postcolonial* (Durham, N.C.: Duke University Press, 2010); Luca Vercelloni, *The Invention of Taste: A Cultural Account of Desire, Delight and Disgust in Fashion, Food and Art,* trans. Kate Singleton, Sensory Studies Series (London: Bloomsbury Academic, 2017).

22. Norbert Elias, *The Civilizing Process,* trans. Edmund Jephcott (Malden, Mass.: Blackwell, 2000).

23. See chapter 6 in Menninghaus, *Disgust.*

24. Mary Douglas, *Purity and Danger* (New York: Routledge, 2002).

25. Miller, *Anatomy of Disgust.*

26. Julia Kristeva, *Powers of Horror: An Essay on Abjection* (New York: Columbia University Press, 1982).

27. Sylvia Yanagisako and Carol Delaney, eds., *Naturalizing Power: Essays in Feminist Cultural Analysis* (New York: Routledge, 1994).

28. Anthropological approaches to taboo accept its role in the structuring of society, often upholding the place and power of patriarchal roles. Consult, e.g., David Akin, "Concealment, Confession, and Innovation in Kwaio Women's Taboos," *American Ethnologist* 30, no. 3 (2003): 381–400; Sigmund Freud, *Totem and Taboo,* trans. James Strachey (New York: Norton, 1950); Valerio Valeri, *The Forest of Taboos: Morality, Hunting, and Identity among the Huaulu of the Moluccas* (Madison: University of Wisconsin Press, 2000).

29. Garland Thomson, *Extraordinary Bodies: Figuring Physical Disability in American Culture and Literature*; Emily Martin, *The Woman in the Body: A Cultural Analysis of Reproduction* (Boston: Beacon, 1992); Anne McClintock, *Imperial Leather: Race, Gender, and Sexuality in the Colonial Contest* (New York: Routledge, 1995).

30. Homi Bhabha, *The Location of Culture* (New York: Routledge, 1994); Judith Butler, *Gender Trouble: Feminism and the Subversion of Identity* (New York: Routledge, 1999); Alexandre Kojeve, *Introduction to the Reading of Hegel: Lectures on the "Phenomenology of Spirit,"* trans. James Nichols (Ithaca, N.Y.: Cornell University Press, 1980).

31. Susan Buck-Morss, "Hegel and Haiti," *Critical Inquiry* 26, no. 4 (2000): 821–65.

32. Franz Fanon, *Black Skin, White Masks,* trans. Richard Philcox (New York: Grove, 2008); Richard Jenkins, "Rethinking Ethnicity: Identity, Categorization and Power," *Ethnic and Racial Studies* 17, no. 2 (1994): 197–223.

33. Nancy Ordover, *American Eugenics: Race, Queer Anatomy, and the Science of Nationalism* (Minneapolis: University of Minnesota Press, 2003); Alexandra Stern, *Eugenic Nation: Faults and Frontiers of Better Breeding in Modern America,* American Crossroads 17 (Berkeley: University of California Press, 2005).

34. Susan Lederer, *Flesh and Blood: Organ Transplantation and Blood Transfusion in 20th Century America* (New York: Oxford University Press, 2008); Lesley Sharp, *Strange Harvest: Organ Transplants, Denatured Bodies, and the Transformed Self* (Berkeley: University of California Press, 2006).

35. Nancy Scheper-Hughes, "Parts Unknown: Undercover Ethnography of the Organs-Trafficking World," *Ethnography* 5, no. 1 (2004): 29–73.

36. For classic anthropological approaches to magic and its relationship to healing practices, consult Edward Evan Evans-Pritchard, "The Morphology and Function of Magic: A Comparative Study of Trobriand and Zande Ritual and

Spells," *American Anthropologist* 31, no. 4 (1929): 619–41; Marcel Mauss, *A General Theory of Magic,* The Norton Library (New York: Norton, 1975); W. H. R. Rivers, *Medicine, Magic and Religion* (New York: Routledge, 2001).

37. Celina Callahan-Kapoor, "Difference and Distinction: Diabetic Publics in the U.S./Mexico Borderlands" (PhD diss., University of California, Santa Cruz, 2016).

38. Julie Guthman, *Weighing In: Obesity, Food Justice, and the Limits of Capitalism* (Berkeley: University of California Press, 2011).

39. Benjamin Aldes Wurgaft, "Incensed: Food Smells and Ethnic Tension," *Gastronomica* 6, no. 2 (2006): 57–60.

40. Marilyn Strathern, "No Nature, No Culture: The Hagen Case," in *Nature, Culture and Gender,* ed. Carol MacCormack and Marilyn Strathern (Cambridge: Cambridge University Press, 1980), 174–222.

41. Miller, *Anatomy of Disgust.*

42.    Philip Joseph Deloria, *Playing Indian* (New Haven, Conn.: Yale Univerisity Press, 2007); Eric Lott, *Love and Theft: Blackface Minstrelsy and the American Working Class* (New York: Oxford University Press, 1995); David Roediger, *The Wages of Whiteness: Race and the Making of the American Working Class* (New York: Verso, 1991).

43. Ruth Frankenberg, *Displacing Whiteness: Essays in Social and Cultural Criticism* (Durham, N.C.: Duke University Press, 1997).

44. Jonathan Metzl, *The Protest Psychosis: How Schizophrenia Became a Black Disease* (Boston: Beacon, 2011).

45. Keith Wailoo, *Dying in the City of the Blues: Sickle Cell Anemia and the Politics of Race and Health* (Chapel Hill: University of North Carolina Press, 2001).

46. Adia Benton, *HIV Exceptionalism: Development through Disease in Sierra Leone* (Minneapolis: University of Minnesota Press, 2015); Michael Montoya, *Making the Mexican Diabetic: Race, Science, and the Genetics of Inequality* (Berkeley: University of California Press, 2011).

47. John Hartigan, *Racial Situations: Class Predicaments of Whiteness in Detroit* (Princeton, N.J.: Princeton University Press, 1999).

48. Lise Widding Isaksen, "Toward a Sociology of (Gendered) Disgust: Images of Bodily Decay and the Social Organization of Care Work," *Journal of Family Issues* 23, no. 7 (2002): 791–811.

49. Elana D. Buch, "Senses of Care: Embodying Inequality and Sustaining Personhood in the Home Care of Older Adults in Chicago," *American Ethnologist* 40, no. 4 (2013): 637–50.

50. Elana D. Buch, *Inequalities of Aging: Paradoxes of Independence in American Home Care* (New York: New York University Press, 2018).

51. Maya Hey, "Fermentation and Delicious/Disgusting Narratives," in *Food in Memory and Imagination: Space, Place, and Taste,* ed. Beth Forrest and Greg de St. Maurice (London: Bloomsbury Academic, 2022), 25–38.

52. Gilles Deleuze, "Control and Becoming," in *Negotiations,* trans. Martin Joughin (New York: Columbia University Press, 1995), 169–82.

53. In many studies of medical governance, which are largely indebted to Michel Foucault's work on governmentality and disciplinary institutions, including his 1976 *The History of Sexuality Vol. 1* and 1975 *Discipline and Punish,* the human body is the endpoint of analysis. The human body might be a carrier of disease, but it is only through acting on the human body that disease—primarily viruses and bacteria—can be acted on. Foundational here is David Armstrong's 1995 *New History of Identity,* which focuses on "surveillance medicine" and the human body as a site of governance and subjection: medical institutions define particular kinds of individuals and behaviors as being at risk or risky, and individuals come to accept and inhabit these classifications, providing the individual with a sense of "identity" and simultaneously providing medical institutions and the state the means to manage populations. This conception of medical governance depends on the bureaucratic and abstractive forms of biopolitics that arose in the nineteenth century to oversee urban and colonial populations, which, according to Ian Hacking's 1990 *The Taming of Chance* and Dorothy Porter's 1986 *Health, Civilization and the State* have their foundations in quantitative, statistical forms of prediction and rationalization, and which focus primarily on the human body as the endpoint of analysis.

54. I discuss this perspective at length in Matthew Wolf-Meyer, *Unraveling: Remaking Personhood in a Neurodiverse Age* (Minneapolis: University of Minnesota Press, 2020).

55. Sarah Whitmee, Andy Haines, Chris Beyrer, et al., "Safeguarding Human Health in the Anthropocene Epoch: Report of The Rockefeller Foundation–Lancet Commission on Planetary Health," *The Lancet* 386, no. 10007 (2015): 1973–2028, https://doi.org/10.1016/S0140-6736(15)60901-1.

56. Michel Foucault, *The Birth of Biopolitics: Lectures at the College de France, 1978–1979,* trans. Graham Burchell (New York: Palgrave, 2008).

57. Deleuze, "Control and Becoming."

58. George Monbiot, *Feral: Rewilding the Land, the Sea, and Human Life* (Chicago: University of Chicago Press, 2017); Shiloh R. Krupar, *Hot Spotter's Report: Military Fables of Toxic Waste* (Minneapolis: University of Minnesota Press, 2013).

59. Alfred E. Kahn, *The Economics of Regulation: Principles and Institutions* (Cambridge, Mass.: MIT Press, 1988).

60. Guthman, *Weighing In.*

61. Roddey Reid, *Globalizing Tobacco Control: Anti-Smoking Campaigns in California, France, and Japan* (Bloomington: Indiana University Press, 2005).

62. Anthropological approaches to the political economy of everyday life are diverse but share a basis in the conception of cultural expectations of consumption as shaping attitudes toward the body, labor, and productivity. Two key texts are

Sidney W. Mintz, *Sweetness and Power: The Place of Sugar in Modern History* (New York: Penguin, 1986), Eric R. Wolf, *Pathways of Power: Building an Anthropology of the Modern World* (Berkeley: University of California Press, 2001).

63. David Harvey, *The New Imperialism* (New York: Oxford University, 2005).

64. Ruth Wilson Gilmore, *Golden Gulag: Prisons, Surplus, Crisis, and Opposition in Globalizing California* (Berkeley: University of California Press, 2007); Guthman, *Weighing In.*

65. Ulrich Beck, *Risk Society: Towards a New Modernity* (Thousand Oaks, Calif.: Sage, 1992); Mary Douglas and Aaron Wildavsky, *Risk and Culture: An Essay on the Selection of Technological and Environmental Dangers* (Berkeley: University of California Press, 1983).

66. Jonathan M. Metzl and Anna Kirkland, eds., *Against Health: How Health Became the New Morality* (New York: New York University Press, 2010).

67. Emily Martin, *Flexible Bodies: Tracking Immunity in American Culture— From the Days of Polio to the Age of AIDS* (Boston: Beacon, 1994).

68. Gilles Deleuze and Félix Guattari, *A Thousand Plateaus,* trans. Brian Massumi, vol. 2 of *Capitalism and Schizophrenia* (Minneapolis: University of Minnesota, MN, 1987), 292–94.

69. David Harvey, *The Condition of Postmodernity: An Enquiry into the Origins of Cultural Change* (Malden, Mass.: Blackwell, 1990).

70. Anthropological approaches to scale have worked to show how discourses about bodies shape the experience of bodies and their agencies, which is based in assumptions about the ascriptive power of language and its limits. Consult, e.g., Charles L Briggs, "Theorizing Modernity Conspiratorially: Science, Scale, and the Political Economy of Public Discourse in Explanations of a Cholera Epidemic," *Cultural Anthropology* 31, no. 2 (2007): 164–87; E. Summerson Carr and Michael Lempert, *Scale: Discourse and Dimensions of Social Life* (Berkeley: University of California Press, 2016); Anna Tsing, "On Nonscalability: The Living World Is Not Amenable to Precision-Nested Scales," *Common Knowledge* 18, no. 3 (2012): 505–24.

71. Matthew Wolf-Meyer, *The Slumbering Masses: Sleep, Medicine, and Modern American Life* (Minneapolis: University of Minnesota Press, 2012); Wolf-Meyer, "'Human Nature' and the Biology of Everyday Life," *American Anthropologist* 121, no. 2 (2019): 338–49; Wolf-Meyer, *Unraveling: Remaking Personhood in a Neurodiverse Age* (Minneapolis, MN: University of Minnesota Press, 2020).

72. Richard C. Lewontin, *Biology as Ideology: The Doctrine of DNA* (New York: HarperPerennial, 1992); Roberts, *Fatal Invention.*

73. John Hartigan, *Care of the Species: Races of Corn and the Science of Plant Biodiversity* (Minneapolis: University of Minnesota Press, 2017); Anna Lowenhaupt Tsing, *The Mushroom at the End of the World: On the Possibility of Life in Capitalist Ruins* (Princeton, N.J.: Princeton University Press, 2015).

74. Nicholas Bauch, *A Geography of Digestion: Biotechnology and the Kellogg*

*Cereal Enterprise* (Berkeley: University of California Press, 2017); Howard Markel, *The Kelloggs: The Battling Brothers of Battle Creek* (New York: Pantheon, 2017); Brian C. Wilson, *Dr. John Harvey Kellogg and the Religion of Biologic Living* (Bloomington: Indiana University Press, 2014).

75. Roediger, *Wages of Whiteness.*

76. For a complementary discussion of marginalized health-seekers, consult Joseph Dumit, "Illnesses You Have to Fight to Get: Facts as Forces in Emergent, Uncertain Illnesses," *Social Science & Medicine* 62, no. 3 (2006): 577–90.

77. Deloria, *Playing Indian;* Kolodny, *Lay of the Land.*

78. Metzl and Kirkland, *Against Health*; Porter, *Health, Civilization and the State.*

79. For discussions of world-building and its ethical implications, consult Arturo Escobar, *Designs for the Pluriverse: Radical Interdependence, Autonomy, and the Making of Worlds* (Durham, N.C.: Duke University Press, 2018), and Tsing, *Mushroom at the End of the World.*

80. Raymond L. Williams, *Marxism and Literature* (Oxford: Oxford Univ. Press, 2009); Matthew Wolf-Meyer, "Where Have All Our Naps Gone?, Or Nathaniel Kleitman, the Consolidation of Sleep, and the Historiography of Emergence," *Anthropology of Consciousness* 24, no. 1 (2013): 96–116.

81. Lila Abu-Lughod, "Writing Against Culture," in *Recapturing Anthropology: Working in the Present,* ed. Richard G. Fox (Santa Fe, Calif.: School of American Research Press, 1991), 137–62; Akhil Gupta and James Ferguson, "Beyond 'Culture': Space, Identity, and the Politics of Difference," in *Culture, Power, Place: Explorations in Critical Anthropology,* ed. Akhil Gupta and James Ferguson (Durham, N.C.: Duke University Press, 1997), 33–51; Michel-Rolph Trouillot, *Global Transformations: Anthropology and the Modern World* (New York: Palgrave Macmillan, 2003).

82. Elizabeth Wilson, *Gut Feminism* (Durham, N.C.: Duke University Press, 2015).

## 1. The Excremental

1. John G. Bourke, *On the Border with Crook* (1891; repr. New York: Charles Scribner's Sons, 1980).

2. John G. Bourke, *Scatalogic Rites of All Nations* (Washington, D.C.: Loudermilk, 1891).

3. Roy Porter, *The Greatest Benefit to Mankind: A Medical History of Humanity* (New York: Norton, 1999); Paul Starr, *The Social Transformation of American Medicine* (New York: Basic, 1982).

4. Norman Gevitz, ed., *Other Healers: Unorthodox Medicine in America* (Baltimore, Md.: Johns Hopkins University Press, 1988).

5. Audra Simpson, *Mohawk, Interruptus: Political Life Across the Borders of Settler States* (Durham, N.C.: Duke University Press, 2014); Kimberly TallBear, *Native American DNA: Tribal Belonging and the False Promise of Genetic Science* (Minneapolis: University of Minnesota Press, 2013).

6. Critiques of objectivity point to the situatedness of the observer, showing how the constitution of objectivity as such relied on the construction of a "view from nowhere" that was isomorphic with a transparent whiteness embedded in North Atlantic patriarchy. For discussions, see Karen Barad, *Meeting the Universe Halfway: Quantum Physics and the Entanglement of Matter and Meaning* (Durham, N.C.: Duke University Press, 2007); Lorraine Daston and Peter Galison, *Objectivity* (New York: Zone, 2007); Donna J. Haraway, *Modest_Witness@Second_Millennium.FemaleMan©_Meets_OncoMouse™: Feminism and Technoscienct* (New York: Routledge, 1997).

7. Bourke discusses survivals through *Scatalogical Rites,* most intensively on 433, 461, 463, 466, 467.

8. An exemplary instance of local medical practices and their colonial opposition is Shirley Lindenbaum, *Kuru Sorcery: Disease and Danger in the New Guinea Highlands* (Palo Alto, Calif.: Mayfield, 1979).

9. Bourke, *Scatalogic Rites,* 440.

10. Bourke, 335.

11. Bourke, 258 (personal notes of September 25, 1878, interview with the chiefs of the Northern Cheyenne; Ben Clark, interpreter).

12. Bourke, 254.

13. Bourke, 262 (quoting Gilder, "Schwatka's Search").

14. Bourke, 5–6.

15. Bourke, 6.

16. Bourke, 6.

17. Quoted in Bourke, 10.

18. Quoted in Bourke, 9.

19. Bourke, 40.

20. Bourke, 460.

21. Bourke, 161.

22. Bourke, 241.

23. Bourke, 124.

24. Bourke, 122.

25. Bourke, 125.

26. Bourke, 56.

27. Mikhail Bakhtin, *Rabelais and His World,* trans. Helene Iswolsky (Bloomington: Indiana University Press, 1984).

28. Harvey Cox, *The Feast of Fools: A Theological Essay on Festivity and Fantasy* (Cambridge, Mass.: Harvard University Press, 1969).

29. Bourke, *Scatalogical Rites*, 15.

30. Bourke, 14. Bourke draws inspiration from contemporary folklorists for this claim: "An American superstition may require for its explanation reference to Teutonic mythology, or may be directly associated with the philosophy, monuments, and arts of Hellas. . . . It is, however, now a recognized principle that higher forms can only be comprehended by the help of the lower forms out of which they grew. . . . The only truly scientific habit of mind is that wide and generous spirit of modern research which, without disdain and without indifference, embraces all aspects of human thought, and endeavors in all to find a whole" (W. W. Newell, in *Journal of American Folk-Lore*, January–March, 1889; quoted in Bourke, *Scatalogical Rites*, 433).

31. Bourke, 97.

32. Bourke, 93.

33. Bourke, 12.

34. Bourke, 392.

35. Bourke, 121.

36. Bourke, 27.

37. Bourke, 432.

38. Thomas Trautmann, *Aryans and British India* (Berkeley: University of California Press, 1997).

39. Bourke, *Scatalogic Rites*, 51–52.

40. Bourke, 14.

41. Quoted in Bourke, 241.

42. Bourke, 118 (quoting Schweinfurth, "Heart of Africa").

43. Bourke, 340 (quoting Cameron's 1877 "Across Africa").

44. Bourke, 361.

45. Bourke, 177.

46. Bourke, 146–47.

47. Bourke, 305.

48. Bourke, 330–31.

49. Bourke, 460.

50. This might serve as a form of "primitive accumulation" according to Dominique Laporte, who argues that the first person to realize the fertilizing potential of their waste and decide to barter it as a good product helped to establish early economic forms—which happen to be based in human shit (*History of Shit*, trans. Nadia Benabid [Cambridge, Mass.: MIT Press, 2000]).

51. Bourke, *Scatalogic Rites*, 459.

52. For a history of conceptions of disease etiologies, consult chapter 9 in Porter, *Greatest Benefit to Mankind*.

53. Bourke, *Scatalogic Rites*, 372.

54. Bourke, 277. Elsewhere, Bourke discusses the possibility that the use of

urine as toothpaste has been diffused from a central community in an attempt to explain how the same practice occurs across a seemingly diverse array of racial types (203–4).

55. Bourke, 374.

56. Quoted in Bourke, 32.

57. Bourke, 182.

## Threshold 1

1. William Beaumont, *Experiments and Observations on the Gastric Juice, and the Physiology of Digestion* (Edinburgh: Neill, 1837), 21.

2. Beaumont, 20.

3. Beaumont, 21.

4. Beaumont, 15.

5. Beaumont, 16.

6. Gilles Deleuze and Félix Guattari, *A Thousand Plateaus,* trans. Brian Massumi, vol. 2 of *Capitalism and Schizophrenia* (Minneapolis: University of Minnesota, 1987).

7. This is the foundational break that is ascribed to the advent of modernity, in which nature and civilization (or Society or Culture) are juxtaposed, as if humans, through their ingenuity, could break themselves from their existence in and dependency on the natural world. For a discussion of this, see Bruno Latour, *We Have Never Been Modern,* trans. Catherine Porter (Cambridge, Mass.: Harvard University Press, 1993).

8. Michael Chazan, "Toward a Long Prehistory of Fire," *Current Anthropology* 58, no. S16 (2017): S351–59.

9. Claude Levi-Strauss, *The Raw and the Cooked,* trans. John Weightman and Doreen Weightman, *Mythologiques* 1 (Chicago: University of Chicago Press, 1983).

10. Alternative and complementary forms of medicine have stressed the ways that it escapes regulation as medicine through appeals to its qualities as food or supplements. On this front, see Hans Baer, *Biomedicine and Alternative Healing Systems in America: Issues of Class, Race, Ethnicity and Gender* (Madison: University of Wisconsin Press, 2001); Roberta Bivins, *Alternative Medicine? A History* (New York: Oxford University Press, 2007); Mei Zhan, *Other-Worldly: Making Chinese Medicine in Transnational Frames* (Durham, N.C.: Duke University Press, 2009).

11. Feminist approaches to "nature" have long argued that the deployment of it as a category is a tool of those in power, particularly as a means to denigrate and control those out of power—usually marked by the gendered, raced, and disabled forms of difference. For key texts in this tradition, see Donna Haraway, *Simians,*

*Cyborgs, and Women: The Reinvention of Nature* (New York: Routledge, 1991); Sylvia Yanagisako and Carol Delaney, eds., *Naturalizing Power: Essays in Feminist Cultural Analysis* (New York: Routledge, 1994).

12. Paul Freedman, *American Cuisine* (New York: Liveright, 2019).

13. Two recent examples of such cookbooks include J. J. Johnson and Alexander Smalls, *Between Harlem and Heaven* (New York: Flatiron, 2018), and Sean Sherman and Beth Dooley, *The Sioux Chef's Indigenous Kitchen* (Minneapolis: University of Minnesota Press, 2017).

14. This is a quickly growing literature that incorporates interdisciplinary perspectives across the humanities and social sciences, many of which build on perspectives related to tradition and everyday practice. See, e.g., Monica Bodirsky and Jon Johnson, "Decolonizing Diet: Healing by Reclaiming Traditional Indigenous Foodways," *CuiZine* 1, no. 1 (2008), erudit.org/en/journals/cuizine/1900-v1-n1 -cuizine2503/019373ar/; Kelly Gordon, Adrianne Lickers Xavier, and Hannah Neufeld, "Healthy Roots: Building Capacity through Shared Stories Rooted in Haudenosaunee Knowledge to Promote Indigenous Foodways and Well-Being," *Canadian Food Studies* 5, no. 2 (2018): 180–95; Annie Lamalice, Thora Martina Hermann, Sébastien Rioux, et al., "Imagined Foodways: Social and Spatial Representations of an Inuit Food System in Transition," *Polar Geography* 43, no. 4 (2020): 333–50; Ashanté Reese, *Black Food Geographies: Race, Self-Reliance, and Food Access in Washington, D.C.* (Chapel Hill: University of North Carolina Press, 2019); Chantelle Richmond, Rachel Bezner Kerr, Hannah Neufeld, et al., "Supporting Food Security for Indigenous Families through the Restoration of Indigenous Foodways," *The Canadian Geographer* 65, no. 1 (2021): 97–109; Carolyn Rouse and Janet Hoskins, "Purity, Soul Food, and Sunni Islam: Explorations at the Intersection of Consumption and Resistance," *Cultural Anthropology* 19, no. 2 (2004): 226–49; Edmund Searles, "To Sell or Not to Sell: Country Food Markets and Inuit Identity in Nunavut," *Food and Foodways* 24, no. 3–4 (2016): 194–212; Edmund Searles, "Food and the Making of Modern Inuit Identities," *Food and Foodways* 10, no. 1–2 (2002): 55–78.

15. For discussions of food-as-medicine approaches, see Nancy Chen, *Food, Medicine, and the Quest for Good Health: Nutrition, Medicine, and Culture* (New York: Columbia University Press, 2008); Judith Farquhar, *Appetites: Food and Sex in Post-Socialist China* (Durham, N.C.: Duke University Press, 2002). The critical issue that Chen and Farquhar address is that the line between "medicine" and "food" is a blurry one. In their indeterminacy, food and medicine—or medicine that passes as food—falls into a zone of self-regulation in which the consumer must decide its riskiness and efficacy.

16. Rene Redzepi and David Zilber, *The Noma Guide to Fermentation* (New York: Artisan, 2018).

17. Salla Sariola, "Fermentation in Post-Antibiotic Worlds: Tuning in to Sourdough Workshops in Finland," *Current Anthropology* 62, no. S24 (2021): S388–98.

18. If there is such a thing as "shit studies," it is necessarily interdisciplinary and pulls from across the social sciences and humanities to consider the role all forms of the excremental play in the organization of social life and the development of individual subjectivities. A cursory bibliography would include Alex Blanchette, "Living Waste and the Labor of Toxic Health on American Factory Farms," *Medical Anthropology Quarterly* 33, no. 1 (2019): 80–100; David Inglis, *A Sociological History of Excretory Experience: Defecatory Manners and Toiletry Technologies* (Lewiston, N.Y.: Mellen, 2000); Dominique Laporte, *History of Shit,* trans. Nadia Benabid (Cambridge, Mass.: MIT Press, 2000); Rachel Lea, "The Shitful Body: Excretion and Control," *Medische Anthropologie* 11, no. 1 (1999): 7–18; Cindy LeCom, "Filthy Bodies, Porous Boundaries: The Politics of Shit in Disability Studies," *Disability Studies Quarterly* 27, no. 1–2 (2007), dsq-sds.org/article/view/11/11; Sjaak van der Geest, "Not Knowing About Defecation," in *On Knowing and Not Knowing in the Anthropology of Medicine,* ed. Roland Littlewood (Walnut Creek, Calif.: Left Coast, 2007), 75–86.

19. For discussions of the promises and perils of bioprospecting, see Cori Hayden, *When Nature Goes Public: The Making and Unmaking of Bioprospecting in Mexico* (Princeton, N.J.: Princeton University Press, 2003); Ayo Wahlberg, "Pathways to Plausibility: When Herbs Become Pills," *BioSocieties* 3, no. 1 (2008): 37–56.

## 2. The Rise of the American Diet

1. Howard Markel, *The Kelloggs: The Battling Brothers of Battle Creek* (New York: Pantheon, 2017).

2. John Harvey Kellogg, *The Stomach: Its Disorders and How to Cure Them* (Battle Creek, Mich.: Modern Medicine, 1896), 49.

3. John Harvey Kellogg, *Dr. Kellogg's Lectures on Practical Health Topics* (Battle Creek, Mich.: Good Health, 1913), 109–10.

4. Kellogg, *Stomach,* 69.

5. Kellogg, *Dr. Kellogg's Lectures,* 29.

6. John Harvey Kellogg, *Colon Hygiene* (Battle Creek, Mich.: Good Health, 1915), 48.

7. Kellogg, 50.

8. Kellogg, *Dr. Kellogg's Lectures,* 73–74.

9. Kellogg, 101–2.

10. Kellogg, 61–62.

11. Kellogg, 102.

12. John Harvey Kellogg, *The New Dietetics: What to Eat and How* (Battle Creek, Mich.: Modern Medicine, 1921), 225.

13. Kellogg, 225.

14. Kellogg, 627.

15. Kellogg, *Stomach,* 67–68.

16. Kellogg, *New Dietetics,* 42.

17. Kellogg, 116.

18. Kellogg, *Dr. Kellogg's Lectures,* 66.

19. Kellogg, *New Dietetics,* 82–83.

20. Kellogg, *Stomach,* 120–21.

21. Kellogg, *Dr. Kellogg's Lectures,* 23.

22. Kellogg, *New Dietetics,* 224.

23. Kellogg, *Stomach,* 34–35.

24. For a discussion of American eugenics movements and their articulations over the early twentieth century, see Nancy Ordover, *American Eugenics: Race, Queer Anatomy, and the Science of Nationalism* (Minneapolis: University of Minnesota Press, 2003).

25. John Harvey Kellogg, *The Living Temple* (Battle Creek, Mich.: Good Health Publishing Company, 1903), 102.

26. Kellogg, 476.

27. Kellogg, *Colon Hygiene,* 78.

28. Kellogg, *Dr. Kellogg's Lectures,* 42–43.

29. Kellogg, *Colon Hygiene,* 212.

30. Kellogg, *New Dietetics,* 203.

31. Kellogg, 830.

32. Kellogg, *Living Temple,* 430.

33. Kellogg, *Dr. Kellogg's Lectures,* 39.

34. Kellogg, 57.

35. For discussions of the rise of hygienic thinking in the United States in the late nineteenth and early twentieth centuries, see Suellen Hoy, *Chasing Dirt: The American Pursuit of Cleanliness* (Oxford: Oxford University Press, 1996); Juliann Sivulka, *Stronger Than Dirt: A Cultural History of Advertising Personal Hygiene in America, 1875–1940* (Amherst, N.Y.: Humanity, 2001); Vincent Vinikas, *Soft Soap, Hard Sell: American Hygiene in an Age of Advertisement* (Ames: Iowa State University Press, 1992); James C. Whorton, *Nature Cures: The History of Alternative Medicine in America* (Oxford: Oxford University Press, 2002).

36. Kellogg, *Dr. Kellogg's Lectures,* 14–15.

37. Kellogg, 16.

38. Kellogg, 14.

39. Kellogg, 25–26.

40. Kellogg, 33.

41. Charles Rosenberg, ed., *Right Living: An Anglo-American Tradition of Self-Help Medicine and Hygiene* (Baltimore: Johns Hopkins University Press, 2003).

42. Matthew Wolf-Meyer, "The Nature of Sleep," *Comparative Studies in Society and History* 53, no. 4 (2011): 945–70.

### 3. Cultivating the Taste for Whiteness

1. For a history of the Rodale Institute and its role in American environmental and dietary thought, see Andrew N. Case, *The Organic Profit: Rodale and the Making of Marketplace Environmentalism* (Seattle: University of Washington Press, 2018).

2. For a discussion of the changing contours of whiteness based on shifting demands in the U.S. labor market, unionization, and suburbanization, see David R. Roediger, *Working Toward Whiteness: How America's Immigrants Became White: The Strange Journey from Ellis Island to the Suburbs* (New York: Basic, 2018).

3. For two approaches to "tolerance" and its role in the United States and other multicultural societies in the post–World War II period, see Jan Blommaert and Jef Verschueren, *Debating Diversity: Analysing the Discourse of Tolerance* (New York: Routledge, 1998); Wendy Brown, *Regulating Aversion: Tolerance in the Age of Identity and Empire* (Princeton, N.J.: Princeton University Press, 2008).

4. Weston A. Price, *Nutrition and Physical Degeneration,* 8th ed. (La Mesa, Calif.: Price-Pottenger Nutrition Foundation, 2008), 444.

5. John Harvey Kellogg, *The Stomach: Its Disorders and How to Cure Them* (Battle Creek, Mich.: Modern Medicine, 1896), 64.

6. Kellogg, 62.

7. Far from an isolated thinker, Price is representative of a broader approach within dentistry that reflected cultural attitudes toward diet and dental well-being. For a discussion of dentistry's history in the United States, see Alyssa Picard, *Making the American Mouth: Dentists and Public Health in the Twentieth Century* (New Brunswick, N.J.: Rutgers University Press, 2009).

8. Price, *Nutrition,* 439.

9. Price, 451.

10. For an example of early approaches to raw foods diets in the United States, see Charles Garras, ed., *Feasting on Raw Foods* (Emmaus, Pa.: Rodale, 1980).

11. For a broader discussion of Davis and her place in American nutrition, see Catherine Carstairs, "'Our Sickness Record Is a National Disgrace': Adelle Davis, Nutritional Determinism, and the Anxious 1970s," *Journal of the History of Medicine and Allied Sciences* 69, no. 3 (2014): 461–91.

12. Daniel Yergin, "Let's Get Adelle Davis Right," *New York Times,* May 20, 1973, 286.

13. Adelle Davis, *Let's Cook It Right, New Revised Edition* (New York: Harcourt, Brace & World, 1962), 440.

14. For a history of milk's role in American dietary practices, see E. Melanie Dupuis, *Nature's Perfect Food: How Milk Became America's Drink* (New York: New York University Press, 2002).

15. Davis, *Let's Cook It Right,* 438.

16. Davis, 442.

17. Adelle Davis, *Let's Eat Right to Keep Fit* (New York: Harcourt, Brace & World, 1954), 19.

18. For summaries of the history of white flight and its impacts on urban communities, see Steven Gregory, *Black Corona: Race and the Politics of Place in an Urban Community* (Princeton, N.J.: Princeton University Press, 1998); Thomas Sugrue, *The Origins of the Urban Crisis: Race and Inequality in Postwar Detroit* (Princeton, N.J.: Princeton University Press, 1998).

19. Adelle Davis, *Let's Eat Right to Keep Fit, Revised Edition* (London: Unwin, 1976), 232.

20. Adelle Davis, *Let's Stay Healthy,* ed. Ann Gildroy (London: Unwin, 1982), 272.

21. Adelle Davis, *Let's Have Healthy Children, New and Expanded* (New York: Harcourt Brace Jovanovich, 1972), 47.

22. Davis, 364.

23. Davis, 382.

24. Davis, *Let's Eat Right to Keep Fit* (1954), 234.

25. Davis, *Let's Cook It Right, New Revised Edition,* 442.

26. Davis, 441–42.

27. Davis, 441.

28. Davis, *Let's Eat Right to Keep Fit* (1954), 61–62.

29. David Kaiserman, "Introduction," in Sonia Uvezian, *The Book of Yogurt: An International Collection of Recipes,* by (New York: HarperCollins, 1999), ix.

30. Kaiserman, x.

31. Kaiserman, x.

32. Stamen Grigoroff, *Étude Sur Une Lait Fermentée Comestible: Le "Kissélo Mléko" de Bulgarie. Revue Médicale de La Suisse Romande* (Geneva: Librairie de L'Université, 1905).

33. Michaela Michaylova, Svetlana Minkova, Katsunori Kimura, et al., "Isolation and Characterization of Lactobacillus Delbrueckii Ssp. Bulgaricus and Streptococcus Thermophilus from Plants in Bulgaria," *FEMS Microbiology Letters* 269, no. 1 (2007): 160–69.

34. James Trager, *The Foodbook* (New York: Grossman, 1970), 371.

35. For a review of this history, see Kingsley C. Anukam and Gregor Reid, "Probiotics: 100 Years (1907–2007) after Elie Metchnikoff's Observation," in *Communicating Current Research and Educational Topics and Trends in Applied Microbiology,* ed. A. Mendez-Vilas (Bajadoz, Spain: FORMATEX, 2007), 466–74.

36. Gayelord Hauser, *Look Younger, Live Longer* (New York: Farrar, Straus & Giroux, 1950).

37. Maguelonne Toussaint-Samat, *History of Food,* trans. Anthea Bell (Malden, Mass.: Blackwell, 1994), 119.

38. Eleanor Motley Richardson, *Andover: A Century of Change, 1896–1996* (Marceline, Mo.: Walsworth, 1995), 68.

39. Quoted in Bonnie Bossart, "Redirection Put Colombo on Leadership Trail," *Industry,* July 1975.

40. Anonymous, "Colombo Makes Fun and Profits with 'New Look' in Yogurt Business," *Griffin Report,* January 1976, 43.

41. Bernice Kanner, "Cultural Revolution," *New York,* July 18, 1983, 14.

42. Kanner, 14–15.

43. Andy Murray, "Bittersweet Memories: Ex-Colombo Owner Reflects on 75 Years of Yogurt Making," *The Eagle-Tribune,* May 20, 2004, 18.

44. Kanner, "Cultural Revolution," 16.

45. For a discussion of California's health culture and its reliance on forms of experimentalism, see Mei Zhan, *Other-Worldly: Making Chinese Medicine in Transnational Frames* (Durham, N.C.: Duke University Press, 2009)..

46. Kanner, "Cultural Revolution," 14.

47. For a discussion of attempts to overcome the gender gap in yogurt's appeal to men, see Emily Contois, *Diners, Dudes, and Diets: How Gender and Power Collide in Food Media and Culture* (Chapel Hill: University of North Carolina Press, 2020).

48. Murray, "Bittersweet Memories," 18.

49. Murray, 18.

50. Anonymous, "Colombo Makes Fun and Profits," 43.

## Threshold 2

1. robgreenfield.org/biography/.

2. robgreenfield.org/healthyeating1/.

3. ers.usda.gov/data-products/food-access-research-atlas/documentation/.

4. robgreenfield.org/healthyeating2/.

5. robgreenfield.org/healthyeating4/.

6. robgreenfield.org/healthyeating3/.

7. robgreenfield.org/healthyeating4/.

8. robgreenfield.org/healthyeating4./

9. robgreenfield.org/healthyeating1/.

10. robgreenfield.org/healthyeating2/.

11. Whiteness studies have long stressed the interactional quality of whiteness, which moves away from whiteness as a static and unchanging quality and instead focuses attention on how whiteness is enacted as a relation between individuals in a specific social context. These contexts are often shaped by colonialism, class, gender, sexuality, and ableism in ways that imbricate race and ethnicity as just one element in complex interactions. For further examples, see Warwick Anderson, *The Cultivation of Whiteness: Science, Health, and Racial Destiny in Australia* (Durham, N.C.: Duke University Press, 2006); Ruth Frankenberg, *White Women, Race Matters: The Social Construction of Whiteness* (Minneapolis: University of

Minnesota Press, 1993); John Hartigan, *Racial Situations: Class Predicaments of Whiteness in Detroit* (Princeton, N.J.: Princeton University Press, 1999).

12. For a deeper discussion of whiteness and transparency, see Woody Doane, "Rethinking Whiteness Studies," in *White Out: The Continuing Significance of Racism*, ed. Ashley W. Doane and Eduardo Bonilla-Silva (East Sussex: Psychology Press, 2003), 3–18.

13. Such an approach echoes concerns in Black Studies and related fields that situate "respectability" as a key element in the shaping of individual behavior, aiming as it does on the cultivation of sensibilities that reinforce dominant, white concerns about bodily comportment and social interactions. For further discussions, see Margot Dazey, "Rethinking Respectability Politics," *The British Journal of Sociology* 72, no. 3 (2021): 580–93; Fredrick C. Harris, "The Rise of Respectability Politics," *Dissent* 61, no. 1 (2014): 33–37; Michelle Smith, "Affect and Respectability Politics," *Theory & Event* 17, no. 3 (2014): n.p.

14. robgreenfield.org/healthyeating1/.

15. robgreenfield.org/healthyeating2/.

16. robgreenfield.org/healthyeating2/.

17. robgreenfield.org/healthyeating3/.

18. robgreenfield.org/healthyeating1/.

19. robgreenfield.org/healthyeating3/.

20. For a discussion of time and its role in participation in community gardens, see Michael Deflorian, "Refigurative Politics: Understanding the Volatile Participation of Critical Creatives in Community Gardens, Repair Cafés and Clothing Swaps," *Social Movement Studies* 20, no. 3 (2021): 346–63.

21. robgreenfield.org/healthyeating3/.

22. robgreenfield.org/healthyeating2/.

## 4. The Arbitrary Rules of Disgust

1. For anthropological approaches to childrearing, see Kathleen Barlow, "Attachment and Culture in Murik Society: Learning Autonomy and Interdependence through Kinship, Food, and Gender," in *Attachment Reconsidered: Cultural Perspectives on a Western Theory*, ed. Naomi Quinn and Jeanette Marie Mageo (New York: Palgrave Macmillan, 2013), 165–88; Bambi L. Chapin, *Childhood in a Sri Lankan Village: Shaping Hierarchy and Desire* (New Brunswick, N.J.: Rutgers University Press, 2014); Judy DeLoache and Alma Gottlieb, *A World of Babies: Imagined Childcare Guides for Seven Societies* (New York: Cambridge University Press, 2000).

2. For broader considerations of how Spock fits into American history and the development of norms in childrearing, see William Graebner, "The Unstable World of Benjamin Spock: Social Engineering in a Democratic Culture,

1917–1950," *The Journal of American History* 67, no. 3 (1980): 612–29; Julia Grant, *Raising Baby by the Book: The Education of American Mothers* (New Haven, Conn.: Yale University Press, 1998); Thomas Maier, *Dr. Spock: An American Life* (New York: Harcourt & Brace, 1998).

3. Benjamin Spock, *Baby and Child Care* (New York: Pocket Books, 1976), 163.

4. On this front, see Elizabeth Povinelli, *The Empire of Love: Toward a Theory of Intimacy, Genealogy, and Carnality* (Durham, N.C.: Duke University Press, 2006). For Povinelli, intimacy is possible through a shared corporeality and mutual understanding of social role as produced through the intertwined ideologies of historical determination and liberal self-fashioning. Such an approach builds on anthropological approaches to the emotions that accept a more robust breadth of emotional possibility as key to true intimacy, such as Renato Rosaldo, *Culture & Truth: The Remaking of Social Analysis* (Boston: Beacon, 1993).

5. This is catalyzed, infamously, in the psychoanalytically informed approach to autism that ascribes its origins to parenting failures, which has since been discredited. See Bruno Bettelheim, *The Empty Fortress: Infantile Autism and the Birth of the Self* (New York: Free Press, 1967).

6. Spock, *Baby and Child Care*, 316.

7. Spock, 481.

8. Spock, 484.

9. Spock, 132.

10. Spock, 163.

11. Spock, 489.

12. Spock, 513.

13. Spock, 481.

14. This is the psychoanalytic basis of disgust and everyday reactions to it, which lead to both a rejection of the disgust-object and a lingering fascination with it. For further discussions, see Sigmund Freud, *Totem and Taboo,* trans. James Strachey (New York: Norton, 1950); Julia Kristeva, *Powers of Horror: An Essay on Abjection* (New York: Columbia University Press, 1982).

15. Spock, *Baby and Child Care*, 289.

16. Spock, 363.

17. Spock, 473.

18. U.S. Department of Labor, Children's Bureau, *Infant Care* (Washington, D.C.: Government Printing Office, 1926), 42–43.

19. Edward Palmer Thompson, *Customs in Common: Studies in Traditional Popular Culture* (New York: New Press, 1993).

20. I discuss this elsewhere in relation to sleep and its association with diurnal rhythms of everyday life, arguing that a widespread use of nature to explain the organization of society and individual biological experiences amounts to a form of

hegemony based in nature (rather than politics in the strict sense). See Matthew Wolf-Meyer, "Natural Hegemonies: Sleep and the Rhythms of American Capitalism," *Current Anthropology* 52, no. 6 (2011): 876–95.

21. Spock, *Baby and Child Care*, 81.

22. Spock, 3.

23. Ellyn Satter, *Child of Mine: Feeding with Love and Good Sense* (Palo Alto, Calif.: Bull, 1991), 323.

24. Satter, 324.

25. Satter, 320–21.

26. Satter, 332.

27. Kim Bookout and Karen Williams, *The Everything Guide to Potty Training: A Practical Guide to Finding the Best Approach for You and Your Child* (Avon, Mass.: Adams, 2010), 39.

28. Bookout and Williams, 40.

29. Mayim Bialik, *Beyond the Sling: A Real-Life Guide to Raising Confident, Loving Children the Attachment Parenting Way* (New York: Simon & Schuster, 2012), 106.

30. Mayim Bialik, "How to Never Use Diapers," YouTube, September 28, 2018, video, 5:50, youtube.com/watch?v=26PP2ItZbf8.

31. This perspective is widely held and fundamental to modern conceptions of biology, as recounted in Ed Yong, *I Contain Multitudes: The Microbes Within Us and a Grander View of Life* (New York: Ecco, 2016).

32. Matthew Wolf-Meyer, "'Human Nature' and the Biology of Everyday Life," *American Anthropologist* 121, no. 2 (2019): 338–49.

## 5. Normal, Regular, Standard

1. Rachel Lea, "The Shitful Body: Excretion and Control," *Medische Anthropologie* 11, no. 1 (1999): 7–18; Lenore Manderson, *Surface Tensions: Surgery, Bodily Boundaries, and the Social Self* (San Francisco: Left Coast, 2011); Linda Mitteness and Judith C. Barker, "Stigmatizing a 'Normal' Condition: Urinary Incontinence in Late Life," *Medical Anthropology Quarterly* 9, no. 2 (1995): 188–210; Michelle Ramirez, Andrea Altschuler, Carmit McMullen, et al., "I Didn't Feel like I Was a Person Anymore: Realigning Full Adult Personhood after Ostomy Surgery," *Medical Anthropology Quarterly* 28, no. 2 (2014): 242–59; Amy Vidali, "Hysterical Again: The Gastrointestinal Woman in Medical Discourse," *Journal of Medical Humanities* 34 (2013): 33–57.

2. Fernanda C. Lessa, Carolyn V. Gould, and L. Clifford McDonald, "Current Status of Clostridium Difficile Infection Epidemiology," *Clinical Infectious Diseases* 55, no. suppl. 2 (2012): S65–70, https://doi.org/10.1093/cid/cis319.

3. Faith Rohlke and Neil Stollman, "Fecal Microbiota Transplantation in

Relapsing Clostridium Difficile Infection," *Therapeutic Advances in Gastroenterology* 5, no. 6 (2012): 403–20.

4. Lawrence J. Brandt, "Fecal Microbiota Transplantation: Patient and Physician Attitudes," *Clinical Infectious Diseases*, September 18, 2012, doi.org/10.1093/cid/cis812; Jonathan Zipursky, Tivon I. Sidorsky, Carolyn A. Freedman, et al., "Physician Attitudes toward the Use of Fecal Microbiota Transplantation for the Treatment of Recurrent Clostridium Difficile Infection," *Canadian Journal of Gastroenterology & Hepatology* 28, no. 6 (2014): 319–24.

5. NIH-FDA, *Fecal Microbiome Transplantation Workshop* (Washington, D.C.: National Institutes of Health and the Food and Drug Administration, 2013). The quotes included in this chapter are drawn from this set of published transcripts provided by the NIH for the meetings, which were transcribed by a professional transcriptionist. I have made only minor grammatical adjustments to the NIH text for ease of readability.

6. Heather Paxson, "Post-Pasteurian Cultures: The Microbiopolitics of Raw-Milk Cheese in the United States," *Cultural Anthropology* 23, no. 1 (2008): 15–47.

7. Brian M. Forde and Paul W. O'Toole, "Next-Generation Sequencing Technologies and Their Impact on Microbial Genomics," *Briefings in Functional Genomics* 12, no. 5 (2013): 440–53.

8. Khiara M. Bridges, *Reproducing Race: An Ethnography of Pregnancy as a Site of Racialization* (Berkeley: University of California Press, 2011); Joseph Dumit, *Drugs for Life: How Pharmaceutical Companies Define Our Health* (Durham, N.C.: Duke University Press, 2012); Stefan Ecks, "Pharmaceutical Citizenship: Antidepressant Marketing and the Promise of Demarginalization in India," *Anthropology & Medicine* 12, no. 3 (2005): 239–54; Emily Martin, *The Woman in the Body: A Cultural Analysis of Reproduction* (Boston: Beacon Press, 1992); Simon J. Williams, "Sleep and Health: Sociological Reflections on the Dormant Society," *Health* 6, no. 2 (2002): 173–200.

9. For a discussion of "standardization" through food and its reflection of norms about eating, bodies, and society, see Elizabeth Dunn, *Privatizing Poland: Baby Food, Big Business, and the Remaking of Labor* (Ithaca, N.Y.: Cornell University Press, 2004).

10. NIH-FDA, *Fecal Microbiome Transplantation Workshop*, 17.

11. NIH-FDA, 33.

12. E. J. DePeters and L. W. George, "Rumen Transfaunation," *Immunology Letters* 162, no. 2 (2014): 69–76.

13. NIH-FDA, *Fecal Microbiome Transplantation Workshop*, 221.

14. NIH-FDA, 169.

15. NIH-FDA, 85.

16. NIH-FDA, 85.

17. NIH-FDA, 230.

18. NIH-FDA, 300.

19. NIH-FDA, 255.

20. NIH-FDA, 168.

21. NIH-FDA, 299.

22. NIH-FDA, 291.

23. NIH-FDA, 37.

24. NIH-FDA, 140.

25. Bruno Latour, *The Pasteurization of France,* trans. Alan Sheridan (Cambridge, Mass.: Harvard University Press, 1988).

26. Johann Peter Frank, *A System of Complete Medical Police,* trans. E. Vilim (Baltimore, Md.: Johns Hopkins University Press, 1976).

27. Patrick E Carroll, "Medical Police and the History of Public Health," *Medical History* 46, no. 4 (2002): 461–94.

28. Markus Dubber, *The Police Power: Patriarchy and the Foundations of American Government* (New York: Columbia University Press, 2005).

29. Karin Johannisson, "The People's Health: Public Health Policies in Sweden," in *The History of Public Health and the Modern State,* ed. Dorothy Porter (Amsterdam: Rodopi, 1994), 165–82.

30. Elizabeth Fee, "Public Health and the State: The United States," in Porter, *History of Public Health,* 224–75; Charles Rosenberg, *Cholera Years: The United States in 1832, 1849, and 1866* (Chicago: University of Chicago Press, 1987).

31. For histories of the CDC and FDA, see Elizabeth W. Etheridge, *Sentinel for Health: A History of the Centers for Disease Control* (Berkeley: University of California Press, 1992); Philip J. Hitts, *Protecting America's Health: The FDA, Business, and One Hundred Years of Regulation* (Chapel Hill: University of North Carolina Press, 2004).

32. Mona Markus, "A Treatment for the Disease: Criminal HIV Transmission/Exposure Law," *Nova Law Review* 23, no. 3 (1999): 847–79.

33. Frank, *System of Complete Medical Police,* 440.

34. Frank, 190.

35. Frank, 142.

36. J. H. Powell, *Bring Out Your Dead: The Great Plague of Yellow Fever in Philadelphia in 1793* (Philadelphia: University of Pennsylvania Press, 1993).

37. Amber Benezra, *Gut Anthro: An Experiment in Thinking with Microbes* (Minneapolis: University of Minnesota Press, 2023); Jamie Lorimer, *The Probiotic Planet: Using Life to Manage Life* (Minneapolis: University of Minnesota Press, 2020).

38. For discussions of how ecologies are managed to produce "clean" spaces, particularly in relation to the promotion of health, see Gregg Mitman, *Breathing Space: How Allergies Shape Our Lives and Landscapes* (New Haven, Conn.: Yale University Press, 2007); Linda Nash, *Inescapable Ecologies: A History of Environment, Disease and Knowledge* (Berkeley: University of California Press, 2006).

39. https://www.rebiotix.com/our-therapy/the-future-of-microbiome-based -therapeutics/; accessed April 6, 2022.

## Threshold 3

1. Lindsey Parsons, "Fecal Transplants and Bipolar Disorder: One Miraculous Recovery That Spurred Many More," *The Perfect Stool,* May 13, 2021, high-deserthealthcoaching.com/fecal-transplants-and-bipolar-disorder-one-miracu lous-recovery-that-spurred-many-more/.

2. For discussions of kind of brains and the molecular powers they have over the actions of individuals, see Joseph Dumit, *Picturing Personhood: Brainscans and Biomedical Identity* (Princeton, N.J.: Princeton University Press, 2003); Emily Martin, *Bipolar Expeditions: Mania and Depression in American Culture* (Princeton, N.J.: Princeton University Press, 2007); Jonathan Metzl, *The Protest Psychosis: How Schizophrenia Became a Black Disease* (Boston, Mass.: Beacon, 2011); Oliver Rollins, *Conviction: The Making and Unmaking of the Violent Brain* (Palo Alto, Calif.: Stanford University Press, 2021).

## 6. Being Gutless

1. This is a pseudonym to preserve the anonymity of the people who contributed to that group. I have additionally applied pseudonyms to the contributors to that group to add a layer of privacy, but have otherwise left the content of their posts unchanged (including typos and syntax errors). The Power of Poop, however, is not a pseudonym, as it is a publicly available website.

2. In this chapter, I do not correct the language used on the internet in informal public forums; it is largely readable, and because how people are communicating is as important as what they are communicating, it seems vital to preserve language as presented. I have changed individuals' names and redacted the date of postings, thereby preserving some privacy in the context of publicly available web content.

3. While I fundamentally disagree with both approaches, these provide the basic coordinates of anthropological approaches to kinship: Marshall Sahlins, *What Kinship Is—And Is Not* (Chicago: University of Chicago Press, 2013); David Schneider, *American Kinship: A Cultural Account* (Chicago: University of Chicago Press, 1980).

4. Nilay S. Shah, Michael C. Wang, Priya M. Freaney, et al., "Trends in Gestational Diabetes at First Live Birth by Race and Ethnicity in the US, 2011–2019," *Journal of the American Medical Association* 326, no. 7 (2021): 660–69.

5. Asher J. Schranz, Jessica Barrett, Christopher B. Hurt, et al., "Challenges Facing a Rural Opioid Epidemic: Treatment and Prevention of HIV and Hepatitis C," *Current HIV/AIDS Reports* 15 (2018): 245–54.

6. For a review of the structural influences of health outcomes, see Jonathan Metzl and Helena Hansen, "Structural Competency: Theorizing a New Medical Engagement with Stigma and Inequality," *Social Science & Medicine* 103 (2014): 126–33.

7. Brooke C. Wilson, Tommi Vatanen, Wayne S, Cutfield, and Justin Martin O'Sullivan, "The Super-Donor Phenomenon in Fecal Microbiota Transplantation," *Frontiers in Cellular and Infection Microbiology* 9, no. 2 (2019): 1–11.

8. Wilson et al., 5–6.

9. Wilson et al., 7.

10. Wilson et al., 6.

11. Katri Korpela, "Impact of Delivery Mode on Infant Gut Microbiota," *Annals of Nutrition and Metabolism* 77, no. S3 (2021): 11–19.

12. Jessica R. Jones, Michael D. Kogan, Gopal K. Singh, et al., "Factors Associated with Exclusive Breastfeeding in the United States," *Pediatrics* 128, no. 6 (2011): 1117–25.

13. Lawrence J. Brandt, "Fecal Microbiota Transplantation: Patient and Physician Attitudes," *Clinical Infectious Diseases,* September 18, 2012, doi.org/10.1093/cid/cis812.

14. Sylvie McCracken, *The SIBO Solutions* (San Bernardino, Calif.: Hollywood Homestead, 2015), 15.

15. McCracken, 77–85.

16. Natasha Campbell-McBride, *Gut and Psychology Syndrome* (Cambridge, UK: Medinform, 2010).

17. For a discussion of the paleo diet and its cultural contours, see Adrienne Rose Johnson, "The Paleo Diet and the American Weight Loss Utopia, 1975–2014," *Utopian Studies* 26, no. 1 (2015): 101–24.

18. Hillary Boynton and Mary G. Brackett, *The Heal Your Gut Cookbook: Nutrient-Dense Recipes for Intestinal Health Using the GAPS Diet* (White River Junction, Vt.: Chelsea Green, 2014).

19. Boynton and Brackett, xiv.

20. Campbell-McBride, *Gut and Psychology Syndrome,* 105.

21. There is voluminous literature on care and caring institutions, most of which points to inequalities in care for care providers and caregivers. Ideally, though, caring institutions might be predicated on a foundation of shared care and the protection of laborers and recipients of care. For a discussion of the possibilities of care, see Heike Drotbohm, "Care Beyond Repair," in *Oxford Research Encyclopedia of Anthropology,* ed. Mark Aldenderfer (New York: Oxford University Press, 2022); Berenice Fisher and Joan Tronto, "Toward a Feminist Theory of Caring," in *Circles of Care: Work and Identity in Women's Lives,* ed. Emily Abel and Margaret Nelson (Albany: State University of New York Press, 1990), 36–54.

## 7. Planetary Health, Scalar Bodies, and the Impossible Turn to Microbial Medicine

1. Thomas Malthus, *An Essay on the Principle of Population,* The World's Classics (Oxford: Oxford University Press, 1993).

2. Sarah Whitmee, Andy Haines, Chris Beyrer, et al., *Safeguarding Human Health in the Anthropocene Epoch: Report of The Rockefeller Foundation–Lancet Commission on Planetary Health,* published in *The Lancet* 386, no. 10007 (2015): 1973–2028, thelancet.com/journals/lancet/article/PIIS0140-6736(15)60901 -1/fulltext.

3. Whitmee et al., 1997.

4. Adia Benton, *HIV Exceptionalism: Development through Disease in Sierra Leone* (Minneapolis: University of Minnesota Press, 2015); Emily Yates-Doerr, *The Weight of Obesity: Hunger and Global Health in Postwar Guatemala* (Berkeley: University of California Press, 2015).

5. Whitmee et al., *Safeguarding Human Health,* 2007–8.

6. Sidney Mintz, *Sweetness and Power* (New York: Penguin, 1985); Eric R. Wolf, *Europe and the People without History* (Berkeley: University of California Press, 1982).

7. Agustin Fuentes, Jonathan Marks, Tim Ingold, and Robert Sussman, "On Nature and the Human," *American Anthropologist* 112, no. 4 (2010): 512–21.

8. Roberto Barrios, "Resilience: A Commentary from the Vantage Point of Anthropology," *Annals of Anthropological Practice* 40, no. 1 (2016): 28–38.

9. Whitmee et al., *Safeguarding Human Health,* 2014.

10. Joel Robbins, "Beyond the Suffering Subject: Toward an Anthropology of the Good," *Journal of the Royal Anthropological Institute* 19, no. 3 (2013): 447–62.

11. Arthur Kleinman, Veena Das, and Margaret Lock, eds., *Social Suffering* (Berkeley: University of California Press, 1997).

12. Miriam Iris Ticktin, *Casualties of Care: Immigration and the Politics of Humanitarianism in France* (Berkeley: University of California Press, 2011).

13. Whitmee et al., *Safeguarding Human Health,* 1987.

14. Whitmee et al., 1992.

15. John Hartigan, *Racial Situations: Class Predicaments of Whiteness in Detroit* (Princeton, N.J.: Princeton University Press, 1999); Karen Ho, *Liquidated: An Ethnography of Wall Street* (Durham, N.C.: Duke University Press, 2009); Hoon Song, *Pigeon Trouble: Bestiary Biopolitics in a Deindustrialized America* (Philadelphia: University of Pennsylvania Press, 2010).

16. Walter Willett, Johan Rockström, Brent Loken, et al., *Food in the Anthropocene: The EAT–Lancet Commission on Healthy Diets from Sustainable Food Systems,* published in *The Lancet* 393, no. 10170 (2019): 447–92, doi.org/10.1016/ S0140-6736(18)31788-4.

17. EAT-Lancet Commission, *EAT-Lancet Commission Summary Report,* 2019, eatforum.org/content/uploads/2019/07/EAT-Lancet_Commission_Summary_Report.pdf, 5, 7.

18. EAT-Lancet Commission, 14.

19. EAT-Lancet Commission, 10.

20. EAT-Lancet Commission, 20.

21. Jamie Snook, Ashlee Cunsolo, David Borish, et al., "'We're Made Criminals Just to Eat off the Land': Colonial Wildlife Management and Repercussions on Inuit Well-Being," *Sustainability* 12, no. 19 (2020), doi.org/10.3390/su12198177.

22. One site where this occurs is in the sensorial reaction to the other, particularly through smell. "Foul" smells index fundamental forms of difference, which are experienced viscerally as a form of disgust. See Constance Classen, "The Odor of the Other: Olfactory Symbolism and Cultural Categories," *Ethos* 20, no. 2 (1992): 133–66; Alain Corbin, *The Foul and the Fragrant: Odor and the French Social Imagination* (Cambridge, Mass.: Harvard University Press, 1986).

23. There is compelling work on the fringes of biomedicine and its encounters with forms of life as therapeutics. See, e.g., Amber Benezra, Joseph DeStefano, and Jeffrey Gordon, "Anthropology of Microbes," *Proceedings of the National Academy of Sciences of the United States of America* 109, no. 17 (2012): 6378–81; Rijul Kochhar, "The Virus in the Rivers: Histories and Antibiotic Afterlives of the Bacteriophage at the Sangam in Allahabad," *Notes and Records of the Royal Society* 74 (2020): 625–51; Jamie Lorimer, *The Probiotic Planet: Using Life to Manage Life* (Minneapolis: University of Minnesota Press, 2020).

# Index

**Matthew J. Wolf-Meyer** is professor in the Department of Science and Technology Studies at Rensselaer Polytechnic University. He is author of *The Slumbering Masses: Sleep, Medicine, and Modern American Life*; *Theory for the World to Come: Speculative Fiction and Apocalyptic Anthropology*; and *Unraveling: Remaking Personhood in a Neurodiverse Age,* as well as coeditor of *Naked Fieldnotes: A Rough Guide to Ethnographic Writing,* all published by the University of Minnesota Press.

Printed and bound by CPI Group (UK) Ltd, Croydon, CR0 4YY

27/10/2024

14581301-0002